QUALITATIVE RESEARCH

Qualitative Research

Studying How Things Work

ROBERT E. STAKE

THE GUILFORD PRESS
New York   London

© 2010 The Guilford Press
A Division of Guilford Publications, Inc.
72 Spring Street, New York, NY 10012
www.guilford.com

Printed in the United States of America

This book is printed on acid-free paper.

Last digit is print number: 9   8   7   6   5   4   3   2   1

Library of Congress Cataloging-in-Publication Data
Stake, Robert E.
    Qualitative research : studying how things work / Robert E. Stake.
        p. cm.
    Includes bibliographical references and index.
    ISBN 978-1-60623-545-4 (pbk.: alk. paper) — ISBN 978-1-60623-546-1
(cloth: alk. paper)
    1. Qualitative research.   2. Research—Methodology.   I. Title.
    H62.S737 2010
    001.4′2—dc22
                                                        2009044464

Acknowledgments

I think they say it takes a village to raise a book. Maybe I don't have that quite right, but these I name here are some of the good people in my village. I thank them for helping me in special ways to make this book good for your experiential knowing.

To my graduate students since 2005, who made my old seem young and who encouraged me to find better ways of explaining why issues are important as conceptual structure for qualitative research.

To C. Deborah Laughton, who treated the writing dear.

To Iván Jorrín Abellán, who saw the art of it.

To Gordon Hoke, who brought themes from far and wide.

To Terry Denny, who came home to get me to going.

To Lizanne DeStefano, who protected the castle.

To Stephen Kemmis, who helped get the book off the ground.

To April Munson, who helped turn outlines into boxes.

To Luisa Rosu, who helped turn workables into patches.

To Rita Davis, who knew how I needed to say it.

To Deb Gilman, who corralled the bibliography.

To Susan Bruce, who pled for permissions.

To kith and kin, as **Tom Hastings** put it.

To all who nudged thoughts and loaned words, lately: **Ivan Brady, Holly Brevig, Rae Clementz, Joy Conlon, Norman Denzin, Svitlana Efimova, Frederick Erickson, Bent Flyvbjerg, Rita Frerichs, David Hamilton, Ernie House, Brinda Jegatheesan, Stephen Kemmis, Sarah Klaus, Eva Koncaková, Saville Kushner, You-Jin Lee, Robert Louisell, Linda Mabry, Barry MacDonald, Ivanete Maciente, Robin McTaggart, Juny Montoya Vargas, Chip Reichardt, Michael Scriven, Thomas Seals, Walênia Silva, Helen Simons, Natalia Sofiy,** and **Terry Solomonson.**

To other reviewers **Silvia Bettez, Janet Usinger, and Deborah Ceglowski,** for their helpful comments.

And, most of all:

To **Bernadine Evans,** who made the experience possible.

Contents

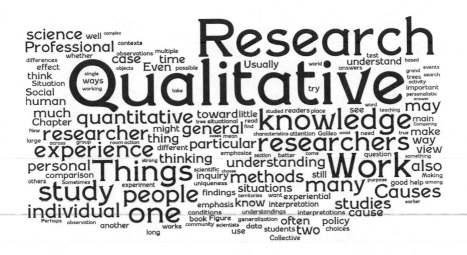

Introduction
Make Yourself Comfortable

In writing this book, I wanted to help create good teaching and learning situations. I wanted to make your class or your reading a better experience. There is much more to teaching and learning than a good textbook, but the experience is better if the book nestles into what you are trying to do. Of course, other teachers and learners are different from you, so this book will nestle with some better than others.

If you are an instructor, you have your content to teach, teaching the way you want to teach, some with lectures—perhaps PowerPointed, maybe with clickers—and maybe small-group discussions. Possibly some blended, maybe all of it online. Were we closer together, I could have written the book better for you. There is content here that needs your explanation, as well as mine. I have built in lots of chocks (a tying place on a boat) for tying in your explanations and examples and questions for the students. I hope you like to assign them large projects, because I think that what I have written becomes more meaningful when projects are being worked on. I have tried to write this book with you in mind—two of us side by side, at safe and reasonable speeds.

If you are a student, you are committing yourself to learning quite a bit more about qualitative research methods. You already know quite a bit. It hasn't been proven yet whether your learning of these things began at conception or at birth, but it really starts early. And it never ends.

Some of what you will want to know will arrive through still-to-happen personal experiences. Like interviewing. You have been asking questions all your life, but for research projects, you probably need to be more disciplined—not necessarily more formal, but more tied into the themes of your study. You can read about it in these chapters and in other writings, but your skill at research interviewing will increase as you do it for real. You need to study and practice, practice and study, back and forth. For that reason, I hope you will be working on a research project while you are reading this book.

If you are a lone reader, pretty much on your own, without instructor and classmates, I feel bad about it, because a lot of this learning is a social experience. And a shared hot chocolate lubricates the mind better than one solo. (As you see, my style here is to try to engage you personally. I know it doesn't always work. I, too, am still trying to figure out how things work.)

This book is about how an understanding of the social and professional worlds around us comes from paying attention to what people are doing and what they are saying. Some of what they do and say is unproductive and silly, but we need to know that, too. A lot of what people do is motivated by their love for their families and a desire to help people, and we need to know that, too. We won't just ask them. We will look closely to see how their productivity and love are manifested.

I put "Studying How Things Work" in the title, not intending to lead you to how things ought to work nor to what factors cause them to work as they do, but intending to help you improve your ability to examine how things are working. Most of the things I have in mind are small things—small but not simple, such as classrooms and offices and committees. But also gerundial things, nursing and mainstreaming and fund-raising, in particular situations. And some special things, such as ordering chairs for a classroom, and "labor and delivery," and personal privacy. Usually, we here will dig into how something particular is working somewhere much more often than into how things work in general. Working toward broad generalizations requires broad studies, most of which need both qualitative and quantitative methods. A dissertation can be a broad study; not all are. What qualitative studies are best at is examining the actual, ongoing ways that persons or organizations are doing their thing.

In writing this book, I chose to emphasize understanding what is currently happening much more than improving what is happening. I am aware that quite a few of you have had your fill of what is happening and want to waste no more time before trying to make things work better. Quite a bit of qualitative research is directed at the problems of professional practice. It looks at poverty and discrimination and standardized testing, and those are good problems for critical study. All of them are complex problems capable of being interpreted differently in different situations. I fear that the problems will be treated superficially if the complexities are not understood. We can speak out against the problem while we are doing the research, but taking an early position for a particular remedy sometimes steers the research away from important insights. You have to do it your way, but the chapters to follow will beg for your patience while you become more expert on how the thing works.

My intention in writing this book is to arrange an experience for you with qualitative research. I care a lot about the words we choose and the methods we use, but it is expanding your experiential knowledge that I prioritize here. Reading, talking, visualizing, being skeptical, working on projects, reflecting—these are important experiences this book will help you with. You will build new ways on top of the ways you already use to figure out how things work. (It is not my intent to make people as much alike as possible. You will run into my skepticism about standardization in the pages ahead.) The grand experience here is contemplating research—not so much handling data, which is important, but thinking through a study from beginning to end.

Your experiences with this book depend, of course, on the words and concepts. To build the experience, I urge you to read right through the unfamiliar words. Otherwise, they may get in the way of the bigger concepts. Hasn't it worked for you all your life? When you need it, there is a glossary just before the bibliography.

The concepts of this book are shaped by my many years as an educational program evaluator. I started my professional career long ago as a teacher, instructional researcher, and developer of educational tests. I found that my quantitative methods failed to answer too many of the questions of program developers and training specialists, so gradually I changed emphasis toward qualitative research methods. I continue to mix quantitative thinking into my designs, but, over the weeks and years, maybe 90% of my research and teaching has emphasized detailed activities of people, experiential inquiry, and close attention to the context of the action. I try to avoid stereotypes, and this includes how I think about you and myself.

PROJECTS

Here are several projects that should help you try out some of the concepts and methods of the dozen chapters ahead.

Project A

From now on, if you do not already do so, keep a journal. It is an extremely important project for you as a qualitative researcher. Make it partly a record of what is happening to your thinking—observations, references, and personal musings—as you experience them. Keep anything worth writing down, stuff like e-mail addresses and book titles. You should start now and carry the journal (laptops don't whip out as easily) with you. From time to time, when an idea is particularly provocative, develop it into a paragraph or more, perhaps making an assertion. You are writing for yourself for now, but you will use some of what you write, later, for others.

Project B

Read at least one classic book by a qualitative writer. Think about what the writer has done to be able to write it. Think about planning, access, fieldwork, distractions, triangulation, barriers to writing. Here are some books that I think of as classics:

Henry Adams: *The Education of Henry Adams* (autobiography)
Howard Becker: *Boys in White* (medical school)
Ronald Blythe: *Akenfield* (English village)
Bruce Chatwin: *The Songlines* (aboriginal territories)
Robert Coles: *Children of Crisis* (urban education)
Ivan Doig: *Winter Brothers* (social expansion of the Northwest)
Mitchell Duneier: *Slim's Table* (poor black men)
Elizabeth Eddy: *Becoming a Teacher* (teacher education)
Robert Edgerton: *Cloak of Competence* (special education)
David Halberstam: *The Coldest Winter* (the Korean War)
Jonathan Harr: *A Civil Action* (legal activism)
Diana Kelly-Byrne: *A Child's Play Life* (preschools)
A. L. Kennedy: *On Bullfighting* (cultural values)
Jonathan Kozol: *Savage Inequalities* (urban schools)
Saville Kushner: *A Musical Education* (a conservatoire)

Halldor Laxness: *Under the Glacier* (church administration)
Oscar Lewis: *La Vida* (a Mexican family)
Elliot Liebow: *Tally's Corner* (gangs)
Sarah Lightfoot: *The Good High School* (portraiture of education)
Barry MacDonald and Saville Kushner: *Bread and Dreams* (school deseg-
    regation)
John McPhee: *The Headmaster* (biography)
Alan Peshkin: *God's Choice* (community and education)
Eric Redman: *The Dance of Legislation* (federal lawmaking)
Margit Rowell: *Brancusi vs. United States* (defining art)
Louis Smith and William Geoffrey: *Complexities of an Urban Classroom*
    (teaching)
Studs Terkel: *Working* (interviews with working people)
James Watson: *The Double Helix* (scientific discovery)
Harry Wolcott: *The Man in the Principal's Office: An Ethnography* (man-
    agement)

Examine the conceptual structure of the book you choose. Consider
what cannot be learned about the conceptual structure of the research
behind the book from what is reported. Note tactics of writing that you
might refer to in the future. Write about it in your journal.

Project C

After reading "The Case of the Missing Chairs" (Box 2.1), go back over
it and look for bias that David Hamilton, the researcher, might have had.
Write a few paragraphs about that possible bias. Put your writing away
until you have read Section 9.4 on bias. Then write another few paragraphs reviewing your original analysis of Hamilton's possible bias.

Project D

Make an observation of at least 3 hours of a large, organized social
event (e.g., a family reunion, a festival, a memorial service, a workshop)
of professional interest to you. If you cannot observe the entire event,
figure out how to learn what happened when you were not there. Learn
as much as you can about the planning and running of it. Presume that
your report might be used to help people far away understand what happened. Identify one or more issues of concern. Discuss this activity and
its issues with someone. Prepare a report, perhaps of 1,000 words.

Project E

After reflecting on Project D (perhaps using no more than a single page), generate at least six rules or reminders for making such a field observation suitable for inclusion in a larger report. Show in the way you write it that you have given it some reflection.

Project F

View the feature-length 2003 film *Kitchen Stories*. What is the message about personal relationships between researchers and the people they study?

Project G

In small groups, discuss: Why should the three items at the end of Section 5.4 be combined into a single score? And why should they not?

Project H

Read Chapter 5 and become familiar with the National Youth Sports Program (NYSP) as it was at the time. Suppose that one of the research team members returns from Metropolis Campus, one of the host campuses, and submits a summary of the program there (Table I.1). The team members get together to decide how this report fits with the other information about NYSP presented in Chapter 5. Study this information, then meet in a small group and talk about what should be done. Prepare a one-page report to the director of the evaluation project, suggesting what should be done.

Project J

Prepare a brief proposal, but at least 800 words long, for carrying out a qualitative research project on a topic of high interest to you. State carefully the research question, one or two issues or additional foreshadowing questions, the relevant contexts, the data to be gathered, the sources from which they will be gathered, other research activities anticipated, two or three most relevant writings that you may build from, the schedule, and the budget. Think carefully about the information most needed by your advisor or host.

TABLE I.1. Summary of the National Youth Sports Program at Metropolis Campus

Prespecified characteristics	Need	Rating	Weight	Merit points
Youth and children				
Quality of experience for youth	High	8	8	64
Knowledge gained by youth				
Sports	Moderate	3	6	18
Personal health	High	3	7	21
Campus/community	Moderate	6	6	36
Staff				
Competence for tasks assigned	High	4	6	24
Dedication, loyalty of staff	High	9	4	36
Quality of staff–student interaction	High	8	9	72
Commitment to structure, discipline	Moderate	9	7	63
Management				
Coordination of activities	High	6	8	48
Compliance with NYSP regulations	High	8	4	32
Responsive to sponsors, parents	High	7	5	35
Coping with emergencies	High	8	6	48
Staff development, supervision	Moderate	3	5	15
Involving staff in management	Low	3	4	12
Attention to kids with special needs	Moderate	5	5	25
Dealing with supplemental costs	Moderate	7	3	21
Bookkeeping	Moderate	6	3	18
Totals			96	588

Note. Ratings scaled 0–10, with 10 high. The summary evaluation score for Metropolis Campus was 588. With the scores of all 170 programs as the reference group, Metropolis Campus scored at the 45th percentile and was identified with 84 other programs in a group called "Commendable with opportunity for enhancement."

Project K

Spend maybe less than an hour sketching out two concept maps, one on "community of practice" and one on "old boys' network" (or two other multiple-reality concepts). Then write a short essay on similarities and differences between the two concepts.

Project L

Write out a qualitative research question of interest to you. Construct five questions that will become part of an interview of one key person to further your understanding of or an assertion about the research question. Presume that it is not his or her feelings or opinions that you need but that his or her experience, observations, or relationships should help you understand. One of the five should be an exhibit question. Think very carefully as you develop the five questions that should try to make the issue more understandable, possibly leading to some resolution of an issue. Presume that other questions will be added later to describe the interviewee as a key person. Think of possible responses by the interviewee and how you would probe them. Try out your five questions on a role-playing helper, then revise the questions. When satisfied with the five, interview someone who has pertinent experience or can role-play it. Make a report showing both the questions planned and the questions asked. Reexamine your questions to see what more you could have done to advance understanding of the issue. Write maybe 500 words about your effort, specifying the issue, the questions, and what you learned here about interviewing.

Project M

Suppose you were including the bubble gum experiment, as described in Section 8.2, in a report, and you were told you could include four photographs to help the reader understand this bubble gum patch. Presume that all the photographs have been provided. Which four scenes might you select?

Project N

Find instances in the Ukraine study (Sections 10.2 and 11.2) that exemplify each of the main characteristics of qualitative research that are identified in Box 1.2.

Project P

Write up a vignette from your own observation or interview data. In a brief accompanying note, identify the issue the vignette develops and an assertion that it might help you make.

Project Q

Suppose a researcher had included in his or her report the vignette of Ana and Issam appearing in Section 12.7. The purpose would be to illustrate an issue or assertion. What might the researcher's issue statement be? Write about it in your journal.

Project R

In small groups, discuss the problem of intrusion and permissions described in Sections 12.3, 12.4, and 12.5.

Project S

Here are some troublesome words you should almost never, or at least very seldom ever, use in a formal report—or at least be careful that your usage is not a cliché: *very, never, truly, genuine, lens, share*. Why should you question the use of each of them? Add some more to the list, such as: *surely, always,* and *paradigm*. What about: *because*?

Project T

Prepare a 15-minute presentation to the class on a topic relevant to this course, such as multiple realities, Flyvbjerg's five misunderstandings of case study, or Parlett and Hamilton's concept of progressive focusing. It might be about the obstacles to access you have faced or iterating report topics from patches and a research question (Section 11.1). If you use PowerPoint, consider it bad form to read from the screen. Consider it an opportunity to teach something that you have come to understand.

CHAPTER 1

Qualitative Research
How Things Work

It is commonly said that science tells us how things work and that the more exact sciences, the quantitative sciences, tell us more exactly how things work, and both are true. At least, if *exact* means *exact*.

Science is the collection of grand explanations of things, physical, biological, and sociological. Science is the explanation of how things work in general, across chemistries and solar systems and cultures. And scientific research is quantitative in many ways. By *quantitative* we mean that its thinking relies heavily on linear attributes, measurements, and statistical analysis.

But each of the divisions of science also has a qualitative side, in which personal experience, intuition, and skepticism work alongside each other to help refine the theories and experiments. By *qualitative* we mean that it relies primarily on human perception and understanding.

The history of science is filled with qualitative thinking, such as that of Newton, Curie, and Watson and Crick. Galileo was one of history's greatest scientists. Using the telescope he invented, he made extensive calculations of the movement of the Earth. As Box 1.1 says, he relied on his feelings of confidence and personal awareness of consistency and observation of particular cases to arrive at his explanations. Heresies and eurekas are part of the story. Ancient and modern research are both qualitative and quantitative.

11

BOX 1.1. Galileo's Situation

Galileo's rejection of Aristotle's law of gravity was not based upon observations "across a wide range," and the observations were not "carried out in some numbers." The rejection consisted primarily of a conceptual experiment and later on of a practical one. These experiments, with the benefit of hindsight, are self-evident. Nevertheless, Aristotle's view of gravity dominated scientific inquiry for nearly two thousand years before it was falsified.

In his experimental thinking, Galileo reasoned as follows: If two objects with the same weight are released from the same height at the same time, they will hit the ground simultaneously, having fallen at the same speed. If two objects are then stuck together into one, this object will have double the weight and will, according to the Aristotelian view, therefore fall faster than the two individual objects. This conclusion operated in a counterintuitive way for Galileo. The only way to avoid the contradiction was to eliminate weight as a determinant factor for acceleration in free fall. And that was what Galileo did.

Historians of science continue to discuss whether Galileo actually conducted the famous experiment from the leaning tower of Pisa, or whether it is simply a myth. In any event, Galileo's experimentalism did not involve a large random sample of trials of objects falling from a wide range of randomly selected heights under varying wind conditions, etc., as would be demanded by the thinking of the early Campbell and Giddens. Rather, it was a matter of a single experiment, that is, a case study, if any experiment was conducted at all.

Galileo's view continued to be subjected to doubt, however, and the Aristotelian view was not finally rejected until half a century later, with the invention of the air pump. The air pump made it possible to conduct the ultimate experiment, known by every pupil, whereby a coin or a piece of lead inside a vacuum tube falls with the same speed as a feather. After this experiment, Aristotle's view could be maintained no longer. What is especially worth noting . . . however, is that the matter was settled by an individual case due to the clever choice of the extremes of metal and feather. One might call it a *critical case*: for if Galileo's thesis held for these materials, it could be expected to be valid for all or a large range of materials. Random and large samples were at no time part of this picture. Most creative scientists simply do not work [that] way with this type of problem.

Source: Flyvbjerg (2001, p. 74). Copyright 2001 by Cambridge University Press. Reprinted by permission.

1.1. THE SCIENCE OF THE PARTICULAR

It can be misleading to say that qualitative thinking provides a pedestal or a readiness for quantitative thinking. It is much more. Qualitative thinking is intermixed within all steps of scientific work. Even when millions of calculations are being processed by a supercomputer, checks on the progress and credibility of aggregative enumeration have been programmed into the operation by visionary and skeptical scientists. That is, qualitative interpretation has been programmed in. All scientific thinking is a mixture of quantitative and qualitative thinking. Research on how things work in the grand schemes of knowledge is both a quantitative and a qualitative task (Roth, 2008). Research is inquiry, deliberate study, a seeking to understand.

A lot of the time, people are interested in how things work in particular situations. A clock is a marvelous concoction of gears and levers, which seem to work the same regardless of person or place or the way the wind blows. But the finest clocks from Switzerland did not work well enough at sea for sailors to navigate their ships until, in the 16th century, John Harrison invented a clock for calculating longitude. Later, we needed a timer for short races. And a special one for 3-minute eggs. Even clockwork is situational.

And the more we study human affairs (as contrasted with physical mechanisms), the more we expect that things will work differently in different situations. How a doctor responds to an injury depends on the sequence of events, the resources available, and the triage priorities.

1.2. PROFESSIONAL KNOWLEDGE

Professional work depends on science, but each profession has a separate body of knowledge of its own. Professional knowledge overlaps with but is different from scientific knowledge. Professional knowledge is the lore gained from working with others having similar training and depth of experience. What especially characterizes professional knowledge is focus on the fact that how things work varies with the situation. The doctor, the lawyer, and the agency chief are masters of thinking about the situation, deciding—from observation and inquiry, from training and experience—on which of the rules and theories to draw.

Clinical knowledge is a form of professional knowledge. It is the knowledge gained by a teacher, nurse, counselor, or other engaged in human services through direct experience with those they are trying to help. Usually the clinician is professionally trained and acts according to professional standards and ethics. Clinical research can be qualitative or quantitative or mixed.

Professional and clinical knowledge rely heavily on qualitative inquiry. However refined the instruments used, it is expected that the choices of action will not be mechanically determined but will be reached through interpretation. Those interpretations will depend on the experience of the researcher, the experience of those being studied, and the experience of those to whom information will need to be conveyed. Professional knowledge relies heavily on personal experience, often in an organizational setting.

When we examine the practices of teaching, nursing, and social work, we see that the characteristics of qualitative research fit nicely. Our purpose here is not to separate the knowledge of practice, clinical knowledge, and professional knowledge. For all of them, qualitative inquiry is interpretive, experiential, situational, and personalistic. These characteristics are spelled out further in Box 1.2.

The fact that all research is both quantitative and qualitative does not mean that both are equally prominent in any single research project. Most projects appear to be either qualitative or quantitative. And those studies with emphasis on personal experience in described situations are considered qualitative.

In this book, "studying how things work" does not mean how all things work in general. This is a book on methods to study how human things work in particular situations. Sometimes, we generalize beyond the particular situation, but we concentrate on how things work in certain contexts, at certain times, and with certain people.

More specifically, we consider how things work within the worlds of professional people: educators, trained caregivers, and organizational managers, for example. It is not that their reasoning powers differ from those of scientists and lay people but that the complexity and substance of their reasoning is shared among professional colleagues and not shared widely with many others.

Many people who do qualitative research want to improve how things work. And empathy and advocacy are and should be part of the lifestyle of each researcher. But focusing on doing good can inter-

BOX 1.2. Special Characteristics of Qualitative Study

(The glossary may help.)

1. **It is interpretive.** It keys on the meanings of human affairs as seen from different views.

    Its researchers are comfortable with multiple meanings.

    They respect intuition.

    On-site observers keep some attention free to recognize unexpected developments.

    It acknowledges the fact that findings and reports are researcher–subject interactions.

2. **It is experiential.** It is empirical. It is field oriented.

    It emphasizes observations by participants, what they see more than what they feel.

    It strives to be naturalistic, to neither intervene nor arrange in order to get data.

    Its reporting provides the reader of the report with a vicarious experience.

    It is in tune with the view that reality is a human construction.

3. **It is situational.**

    It is oriented to objects and activities, each in a unique set of contexts.

    It makes the point that each place and time has uniqueness that works against generalization.

    It is holistic more than elementalistic, not reductively analytic.

    Its designs seldom emphasize direct comparisons.

    Its contexts are described in detail.

4. **It is personalistic.** It is empathic, working to understand individual perceptions. It seeks uniqueness more than commonality; it honors diversity.

    It seeks people's points of view, frames of reference, value commitments.

    Often issues are emic (emerging from the people) more than etic (brought by researchers).

    Even in interpretations, there's preference for natural language, disdaining grand constructs.

    The researchers are ethical, avoiding intrusion and risk to human subjects.

    The researcher is often the main research instrument.

(cont.)

BOX 1.2. *(cont.)*

5. **When qualitative study is done well, it is also likely to be . . .**

    . . . **well triangulated,** with key evidence, assertions, and interpretations redundant.

    Before reporting, researchers try deliberately to disconfirm their own interpretations.

    The reports give ample information so readers can make their own interpretations, too.

    The reports assist readers in recognizing the researchers' points of view, subjectivity.

    . . . **well informed** about main theories and professional understandings related to the inquiry.

    Its researchers are methodologically competent and versed in relevant substantive disciplines.

    The reports refer to relevant literature but do not attempt to teach that literature.

6. **Qualitative researchers have strategic choices, leaning more one way or another, toward . . .**

7. aiming at knowledge production or toward assisting practice or policy development.

8. aiming to represent typical cases or toward maximizing understanding of unique cases.

9. advocating a point of view or toward advocacy of a point of view.

10. emphasizing the most logical view or toward laying out multiple realities.

11. working toward generalization or working toward particularization.

12. quitting after providing findings or toward continuing making improvements.

fere with understanding how things work and ultimately may weaken improvements by "blueprinting" the works too simply. Advocacy may endanger research by getting in the way of skepticism (more on this in Chapter 12).

Research enlists different personalities in research. The constituency of a research community needs a variety of personalities. Either too much commitment to change or too much skepticism, across the community, will crimp the scope and zest of research. Each researcher has an obligation to think about activism and reticence and to recognize them in him- or herself—and for the good of community, perhaps welcoming difference in others.

1.3. INDIVIDUAL EXPERIENCE AND COLLECTIVE KNOWLEDGE

At the personal or individual level, we know the ways many things work. We may experience them as episodes in a situation. The tree in my front yard is easy to climb. Also, we know many things collectively, as generalizations across episodes and situations. Collectively, we know that trees easy to climb have low, strong limbs a few feet apart. That's how my tree works. That's how climbing trees in general works. These two pieces of knowledge, the individual and the collective, represent two territories of epistemology (the study of knowledge). One piece is knowledge about particular situations. And the other is about situations in general. When the main aim is to build theories, a respected qualitative way of moving from individual knowledge to collective knowledge is "grounded theory" (Strauss and Corbin, 1990). But in the present book, the main aim is to build individual knowledge.

Another way of referring to knowledge territories in your brain is as generalization and particularization. These two territories can also be thought of, roughly, as inquiry territories, those two territories of science and professional work. Scientists try to find out what is true in general. Professional people try to find out what is true about individual clients, classrooms, or communities. Of course, professionals are also interested in general knowledge. They could not deal effectively with individual situations unless they had lots of understanding of science, tradition, and other general knowledge. And scientists—Galileo, for example—are interested in the individual observation. But their main effort is toward better understanding of general relationships and making better theory. These two territories overlap, but epistemologists have found it useful to think separately about each.

We want to know more about trees than how "climber friendly" they are. We want to know about tree characteristics in general: more than can be experienced about any one tree, more than can be experienced by any one person. Individual knowledge is the knowledge about one thing in its time and in its own place and about how it works. Epistemologically we say that we can embrace the tree. Not just for haptic sensations but to know it personally. It may be important who had the experience. It may not. For generalizations about climber-friendly trees, we may not care where the knowledge came from or whether it is useful or universally true.

That is not all we can know about trees. There is much more than what you have learned yourself. Any generalization about all trees has to be true also for a person in Iceland, where the trees are too short to be climbed.

Two realities exist simultaneously and separately within every human activity. One is the reality of personal experience, and one is the reality of group and societal relationship. The two realities connect, they overlap, they merge, but they are recognizably different. What happens collectively (for a group) is seldom the aggregation of personal experience. Hurricane Katrina was a collective experience for the people of the world, not the sum of the individual experiences inside New Orleans and elsewhere. The assassination of Abraham Lincoln was, first of all, an individual experience for him, not something derived from the shock felt throughout societies. What happens individually is much more than the separation of collective relationships. We can come to understand the particular and thus comprehend a little more the general, but not much. We can try to apply general knowledge in an individual case but with little improvement in understanding that case. Transformation of knowledge from individual to aggregate and back is fraught with fraughtfulness. Both realities exist with some degree of separation.

Sociologists and others sometimes distinguish between macroanalysis and microanalysis.[1] Studies about world cultures and social systems are macroresearch; those about local neighborhoods and individuals are microresearch. Theory building and policy analysis studies using collective knowledge are macroresearch, and studies of the individual are microresearch. The big picture versus the close-up. More often than not, microstudies are qualitative studies. Macrostudies are often based on aggregations of quantitative data. Microstudy tends to go after the individual case. Macrostudy tends to examine large groups at a distance.

We who study human activity constantly encounter macrocosmic and microcosmic views, even of homes and recreation vehicles. In any

---

[1] *Macrocosms* are the big things, the world, or the universe as a whole. *Microcosms* are the small communities or individual people, sometimes representative of the larger things, but often not.

given study, qualitative researchers usually choose to emphasize the micro over the macro. Qualitative researchers usually prefer the close-up view. We researchers take a single case to study, a case unique in some respects, and emphasize the nature of that particular case. Or, following Harvey Sacks (1984), we choose to generalize as to the nature of other cases not studied. We do both, but usually not in the same study.

If researchers choose to gather experiential data more than measurements, they call their research "qualitative"—but they still may emphasize either the particular or the general. If findings are drawn primarily from the aggregate of many individual observations, we call the study "quantitative," but the researcher still may emphasize either the particular or the general. If researchers set formal standards for assessing the findings, we operate closer to the mechanisms of social science, but we still may emphasize either the particular or the general. Researchers use mixed methods (Creswell and Plano Clark, 2006), but most of us are consistent in leaning toward the experiential or the metric. Most of us have our favorite methods, but to some extent, we seek to understand both the individual and the collective.

1.4. THE METHODS OF QUALITATIVE RESEARCH

Our methods are many and widely shared across many research fields, from anthropology to biography to ceramics to zoology. And yet there is no single field in which we find all the methods of qualitative research regularly used. Child study and critical study each have a good tool kit of methods, but writing newspaper editorials and country music also contributes to the grand collection of methods. Within qualitative methods in all fields, you can find the characteristics identified in Box 1.2.

As indicated earlier, the distinction between quantitative and qualitative methods is a matter of emphasis more than a discrete boundary. In each ethnographic, naturalistic, phenomenological, hermeneutic, or holistic study—that is, in each qualitative study—the quantitative ideas of enumeration and recognition of differences in size have a place. And in each statistical survey and controlled experiment—in each quantitative study—natural-language description and researcher interpretation are to be expected (Ercikan and Roth, 2008). Perhaps the most important methodological differences between qualitative and quantitative are twofold: the difference between (1) aiming for explanation and (2) aiming for understanding, and the difference between (1) a personal role and (2) an impersonal role for the researcher. Both will be differences in shading, varying over time, choices usually to be made by the researcher.

What we mean by *explanation* and *understanding* is developed in the next section (and in the early pages of Chapter 3 and in Section 11.4). The difference between roles for the researcher is important—a matter of gradation from impersonal into personal. For qualitative research, as indicated earlier, the researcher him- or herself is an instrument, observing action and contexts, often intentionally playing a subjective role in the study, using his or her own personal experience in making interpretations. The quantitative researcher makes methodological and other choices based partly on personal preference but usually tries to gather data objectively rather than subjectively.

Observation, interviewing, and examination of artifacts (including documents) are the most common methods of qualitative research. We take them up in Chapter 5. It is much the same as when, in the past, you have been satisfying your curiosity, getting acquainted with someone new or shopping for shoes. This book should help you make the methods you use more disciplined and trustworthy. Before we do that, we need to reflect quite a bit more on the meanings of qualitative research—not just the definition, but what that way of inquiry will come to mean to you.

Qualitative research methods are built around experiential understanding, which we take up in Chapter 3. The methods will be different depending on whether particularization or generalization is our orientation. That topic is taken up again in Chapter 11. But well before that, you will have a good sense of the difference between research aimed at understanding a particular situation versus research done to explain situations in general.

1.5. CAUSES

As your author, I approach writing this section with some trepidation. I'm a little scared. It's not that I fear that I will say it wrong. I will do my homework, and I will get wise people to check it. It is not that it is too political and I might get in trouble. It is political, and the federal view (as I started to write this) is that causal research is the "gold standard" and that qualitative research is inferior. But at age 80, I'm safe. It is that

I cannot think of a good way to make this topic one you want to read. Is there anything I can do to cause you to really want to read this section?

It is not that the topic is not useful. Almost everything we do is intended to have an effect. We brush our teeth to protect them. We watch sports to enjoy being connected to our favorite teams (mine is the Chicago Cubs). We send our kids to school to become educated. Cause and effect.

Poet Ralph Waldo Emerson (1850) said, "Shallow men believe in luck. Strong men believe in cause and effect." Many researchers think that the main purpose of science is the search for cause and effect. Some science is not the search for cause and effect (taxonomy, for example)— but much is. Theoretical and applied science, as well as professional thinking—all seek explanations, influences of forces of any kind, including culture, personality, economics. Given effects, we search for causes. Given interventions, we search for effects. We want to explain what makes things work. How can we make health care better? What are trans fats doing to our hearts? How can we lose weight?

Australian philosopher J. L. Mackie (1974) described causation as "the cement of the Universe," meaning that things work because they are caused to work. We usually think that if we know the causes, we can fix what isn't working. But finding causes perplexes not just repair persons; it perplexes scientists and philosophers. It is perplexing partly because causes can be subtle, because they can work differently in different situations, and because people do not agree as to what a cause is.[2] Why didn't my granddaughter complete her assignment? Lack of motivation? Too busy? Enjoys frustrating her elders? Ask her and she says, "I don't know." That probably is true. And we might study her carefully a long time without finding the causes of her putting off her assignments, nor the effects.

Could it be possible that there are no causes for some child behavior? Could it be possible that there are no causes for anything? Are there really explanations for missed assignments, for the failure of a school, for the rise of the national debt? Or are there too many causes to account

---

[2] In his review of this section, quantitative methodologist Charles Reichart chided me for talking so much about seeking causes and so little about seeking effects. He said it is common knowledge that causes will not be found. Searching for effects of a specified cause is what he saw as a more common aim, particularly of program evaluation.

for? It is possible that the cement of the universe may not explain very much. Is that talking nonsense? One of the skeptics was writer Leo Tolstoy. In *War and Peace*, he argued over and over against simplistic identification of causes. He said:

> Why does an apple fall when it is ripe? Is it brought down by the force of gravity? Is it because its stalk withers? Because it is dried by the sun, because it grows too heavy, or the wind shakes it, or because the boy standing under the tree wants to eat it? (1869/1978, p. 719)

There are many conditions that apparently coexist with and possibly contribute to the apple's fall. The influences change with the weather and with the boy's appetite. Even a violent windstorm has to share causality with the condition of the stem.

Philosopher John Stuart Mill said, "If a person eats of a particular dish, and dies in consequence, that is, would not have died if he had not eaten of it, people would be apt to say that eating of that dish was the cause of his death" (1843/1984, Book III, Chapter 5, Section 3). Makes sense. But people also are interested in those mushrooms the cook used. And in the fact that his wife filled and refilled his plate. We do not have to presume that all conditions are equally worth considering. But we may say too little if we speak only of one cause.

Tolstoy said it is wrong to think of main causes, because they promise more than they can deliver—that we are better off looking at the changing conditions. For important human matters, rather than attributing the effect to a couple of main causes, Tolstoy advised us to describe the events as best we can. Some of the events are statements of various people as to what they believe to be the cause. Perhaps the boy rubs his lucky ring while pulling the branch.

Tolstoy's strategy may be all right for him, because his job was to tell the story of Napoleon's invasion of Russia. He was not an advisor to General Kutuzof on how to defend Moscow. Tolstoy did not have to set a policy. In times of impending invasion and at all times, people need to make choices among alternative actions, including the choice not to act at all. We would like to see more choices based on research.

We have basic research that tells us that many things work in general. The findings help us to set a framework for thinking. Usually one basic study goes no further than to tell us some of the more important things to pay attention to. And basic research tells us that nothing works all the time and that many are the possible impediments to success. Experimental methods are good for telling us about small but persistent effects of a specific action across a large number of situations.[3]

Usually, in the study of human affairs, the large-scale, well-monitored cause-seeking experiments are costly—usually well beyond doctoral research resources. In social field studies, controlling the conditions (conditions such as seriousness of participants, using materials in the prescribed manner, obtaining measurements properly) has been very difficult. Most quantitative researchers do straightforward comparison and correlational studies, mixing in some experimentation, paying attention to how conditions, often many conditions, change together. Correlational studies, including causal modeling, contribute little to determination of cause or effect, but they provide suggestions as to how to manage a problem or create a new program (Scriven, 1976).

Qualitative researchers are seldom involved in setting major social policies, but they feel that people who set policy can profit from becoming acquainted with ethnographic, program evaluation, and other qualitative studies. As discussed in Chapter 11, they will claim that with knowledge of the particular action of a family or clinic, for example, the policy setters and practitioners can get a better sense of the important functions in a complex situation, even when it is a situation quite unlike their own. There will be some instances in which readers will think of ways to borrow something technical from a qualitative study, but usually it is expected that the reader gets a greater sense of experience from complex situations.

The qualitative researcher uses some of the words of causal connection, verbs such as *influences, inhibits, facilitates,* and even *causes,* but (if done properly) makes reference to the limited, local, and particular place and time of the activity. Even then, the qualitative researcher usually tries to assure the reader that the purpose has not been to attain generalization but to add situational examples to the readers' experience.

War and Peace is an experiential story of the defeat of Napoleon's army after a deep winter in which the Russian army did not fight, just

---

[3]Many of those who advocate randomized controlled trials (RCTs), with experimental groups compared with control groups, have been impressed by the (great but not universal) success of pharmaceutical science in the past few years. (And they acknowledge the deceit that can occur when the studies are not done properly; see House, 2006; more about the nature of evidence is in Chapter 7.)

stayed out of range. Kutuzof retreated and retreated, avoiding being overwhelmed by the superior French forces. Eventually the French turned around and dragged back home with less than 10% of their soldiers alive, a momentous deterrent to French imperialism. How did it start? We can see Tolstoy at his best dealing with the question "What caused this war, anyway?"

> Although Napoleon at that time, in 1882, was more convinced than ever that to shed or not to shed the blood of his peoples—*verser ou ne pas verser le sang de ses peuples*, as (Tsar) Alexander expressed it in his last letter to him—depended entirely on his will, he had never been more in the grip of those inevitable laws which compelled him, while to himself he seemed to be acting on his own volition, to perform for the world in general—for history—what was destined to be accomplished.
>
> The people of the west moved eastwards to slay their fellow-men. And, by the law of coincidence of causes, thousands of minute causes fitted together and co-ordinated to produce that movement and that war: resentment at the non-observance of the Continental System, the Duke of Oldenburg's wrongs, the advance of troops into Prussia—a measure undertaken (as Napoleon thought) solely for the purpose of securing armed peace—and the French Emperor's passion for war, and the habit of fighting which had grown upon him, coinciding with the inclinations of his people, who were carried away by the grandiose scale of the preparations, and the expenditure on those preparations, and the necessity of recouping that expenditure. Then there was the intoxicating effect of the honours paid to the French Emperor at Dresden, the diplomatic negotiations which in the opinion of contemporaries were conducted with a genuine desire to achieve a peace, though they only inflamed the *amour propre* of both sides, and millions upon millions of other coincident causes that adapted themselves to the fated event. (1869/1978, p. 718)

To be sure, that invasion of Russia was different in magnitude and complexity from the commissioning of a family service center or the decision to send a child to a private school. But all of them have multiple causes, multiple preconditions. And to us making the decision, we recognize the pressures, but we also think we, like Napoleon, are free to choose the action.

The researcher who studies the decision may seek to identify the main cause or the most important causes, but it will not be possible to claim that without that cause, the effect (the commissioning, the decision) would not have happened. The resources needed for research are large, and we would like to promise that we will find causes, but we cannot, neither with certainty nor even with a high degree of confidence.

We seek to understand how something works. Whether we are quantitative or qualitative researchers, we do need to search for causes, for influences, for preconditions, for correspondences. Our findings and stories can enlighten those seeking to understand the history or the problem or seeking to change the policy. But the data, however analyzed, do not themselves resolve the problem. It is the interpretation of the data, of the observations and measurements, that will stand, not as proof but as persuasion of one meaning more than another. We think about causes because it helps discipline our research. But we should keep in mind Tolstoy's obsession with the idea of countless multiple causes.

Still, we work with people who think of simple cause and effect. It is clear to them that things are caused. It seldom will be useful for us to preach to them Tolstoy's religion of multiple concurrences. We should try to minimize overexpectations of causality, but we sometimes have to talk their language.

For the more immediate future, we should edit our sentences carefully to diminish the "attribution to cause." We should not say, "The director terminated the policy because he was upset." but "The director terminated the policy. He said that he was upset." We should not say, "The River Dnieper froze because the temperature dropped below zero Celsius," but "The River Dnieper froze as the temperature dropped below zero Celsius." We should not say, "The disability program was stopped because the bond issue failed," but "After the bond issue failed, the disability program was stopped."—Or is it important to reduce the implications we make about causality? You have to decide. (So, in my view, the section wasn't so boring after all.)

1.6. THE THING

The word *thing* isn't a technical word. But we need it as a technical word for the best use of this book. Let's use the word *thing* to identify the target of the research project. There isn't a technical word for the target, and there needs to be. So what researchers are studying is "the thing." The thing could be an organization, such as an employment bureau or a child-care center. The thing could be a policy, such as a triage policy or a civil rights policy. It could be a relationship between the churches of a community. It could be a phenomenon such as the use of cell phones in rural China. The thing is what is being studied: a person, a family, a riot, a corporate merger. A research project could have more than one thing, or none at all, but most qualitative studies will have *a thing*. The title of the book means: *Qualitative Research: Studying How Things Work.* Keep the word *thing* in mind as you read this book.

The community of researchers encourages each individual researcher to choose what things he or she will study. Of course, if the researcher works for someone else, the researcher will have less choice but, even in the most restrained organizations, will have some opportunity to define the content to be studied. Others may criticize the choices researchers make, but it is generally agreed that research quality depends on giving researchers freedom to decide the things to study.

The benefits of research are not evenly spread among the researcher, the research community, the home institution or corporation, the public, and others. Science and the professions push, sometimes against each other, to have the research benefit them. Policy and practice can be improved by good research and hurt by bad research. Some benefits occur by studying how people feel about things; we may call it survey research or polling. Most social research asks not how people feel but how things work. It often helps to have people report how they see things working, but most good data come from observations researchers make about processes, products, and their artifacts. These ideas about "the thing studied" are developed more in Section 5.2 on interviewing.

1.7. COMPARING THINGS

Science seeks understandings of how things generally work, understandings of causes and effects. That includes functional relationships such as "The higher the emphasis on student performance on test scores, the greater the teaching to the test." One of the most common ways of arriving at such generalizations is to compare things, such as comparing the states having high-stakes testing with states having low-stakes testing as to how much teaching becomes oriented to the content of the standardized achievement tests. One could also, for a number of schools, examine levels of emphasis on test scores and levels of teaching to the test and see how they correlate. One could also do case studies of a few teachers, looking at their perceptions of pressure for increasing test scores and separately looking at how much they depart from the prescribed curriculum guidelines. Both quantitative and qualitative methods can be used to seek a functional relationship.

Of the three methods—comparison, correlation, and case study—the crudest is the comparison. It ignores huge differences within the two groups. Case studies are simplistic in that they look at only one or a few classrooms, but they can look most carefully at levels in test emphasis and teaching. Correlation studies pay attention to gradation but usually give little attention to classroom activities.

Many qualitative researchers make little place for grand comparison (such as between age groups) in their research designs. Still, there is some attention to comparison in almost every interpretation. When we state something, we also think about what else is implied. When we say three people shared a room, we almost cannot avoid a mental comparison as to how crowded it would be with four and how much less interactive it would be with one. We compare how well three fit the room by thinking of what would be going on in the room—practicing drums and using laptops, for example. Comparison is a close companion to description and an essential aid to interpretation—but it is not the strongest basis for coming to understand how a thing works.

Much qualitative research aims at understanding one thing well: one playground, one band, one Weight Watchers group. Or one phenomenon, such as the relationship among siblings as to clothing choices. There will be small comparisons all along the way, but how things work depends mostly on observing broadly how some of the individual things work rather than on comparing one group to another. That is the ordinary way qualitative researchers work. It is consistent with their priorities on uniqueness and on context.

Some researchers study recidivism, that is, breaking the rules again after being punished for breaking them earlier. A qualitative researcher might (1) study a single repeating rule breaker or (2) take a group of rule breakers and closely examine the complexities of their motivation, peer group, and attitudes toward rules. Many new researchers will propose to compare on several criteria a few recidivists with a few who do not repeat the offense. That is a weak design. That comparison might show some differences, possibly statistically significant, but these findings would probably not be as informative of the complex situations as the two designs mentioned earlier. What is the point here? What is weak about comparisons?

Partly because it fits the appetites of advocates and the news media, much of the world news and many scientific findings are based on comparisons. Yesterday's stock market drop. Deaths in refugee camps in the year 2007. Nations compare their educational systems on the basis of standardized tests. It is simplistic, but they do. The United States ranked 28th on one of the Program for International Student Assessment (PISA) tests, an embarrassing comparison (McGaw, 2007). Many more criteria, many more factors, many more stories should be reported, many should be demanded. That amount of U.S. embarrassment might be the right amount, but we should know more than what one indicator tells. Whether the statistic is valid or not, any interpretation based on a single statistic invites invalid interpretations.

Those studies called comparative studies often take a macroperspective, comparing nations or cultures or communities. It is difficult for them to avoid reducing complex differences to stereotypes.

A stereotype is a simplistic representation, often a misrepresentation. It often is remembered after the details are forgotten. When we study the question, How does something work?, we see ways we can simplify the understandings. But we run the danger of simplifying too much. We also run the danger of dwelling on the nuances of complexity too much, making things too difficult to understand. We need to use our methods of qualitative research in ways that avoid both oversimplifying and overcomplicating the understandings for our readers. Panels you create to review your research can be of help.

Qualitative research contributes to stereotyping but also fights against it. By emphasizing a particular experience, dialogue, context, and multiple realities, a researcher can lessen the chance of simplistic understanding. But this researcher also reduces the chance of improving general understandings. Emphasis on comparison may give us what we want most to know, caring little to know about the complexity. Is it possible that by knowing the individual people better, we come to know less about people in general? Perhaps yes, perhaps no. There is a great intuitive power within each of us to generalize. And then we worry, as we do in Chapters 7 and 11, about the quality of our generalizations.

1.8. WEAKNESSES OF QUALITATIVE RESEARCH

Qualitative study has its supporters and disdainers. I am a deeply devoted supporter; yet I have long felt the disappointment of some sponsors and colleagues. The weaknesses are pretty much what the disdainers say they are. Qualitative research is subjective. It is personalistic. Its contributions toward an improved and disciplined science are slow and tendentious. New questions emerge more frequently than new answers. The results pay off little in the advancement of social practice. The ethical risks are substantial. And the cost is high (see Silverman, 2000, p. 9).

Yet the effort among professional people to promote a subjective research paradigm is strong (Lagemann, 2002). Subjectivity is not seen by them (and myself) as a failing, something to be eliminated, but as an essential element of understanding human activity. Yes, understanding will sometimes be misunderstanding, by us researchers and by our readers. Misunderstanding will occur partly because we researcher–interpreters are unaware of our own intellectual shortcomings; also partly because we treat contradictory interpretations as useful data. Qualitative researchers have a respectable concern for validation of observations; we have routines for "triangulation" (see Chapter 7) that approximate in purpose those in the quantitative fields. But we do not have procedural rules and reviews that put subjective misunderstandings to stiff enough a test.

The phenomena being studied by qualitative researchers are often long and episodic and evolving. It often takes a long time to come to understand what is going on, how it all works. The research is labor intensive and the costs are high. For many studies, these are labors of love more than the work of science. Some of the findings are esoteric. The worlds of commerce and social service benefit all too little from these investments. More may come for those who study their own shops and systems by these methods, but too few of them bring the disciplined views of the specialist into play.

These are personal studies. The issues of other human beings quickly become issues of the present research. Privacy is always at risk. Entrapment is regularly a possibility, as the researcher raises questions and options previously not considered by the respondent (see Chapter 12). A tolerable frailty of conduct close among us becomes a questionable ethic in distant narrative. Some of us "go native," accommodating to viewpoint and valuation of the people at the site, then reacting more critically when back again with academic colleagues (Stake, 1986).

Often the gains in perspective are worth these costs. The value of intensive and interpretive study is widely apparent. We remember that for many years the findings were considered unworthy of full respect by many research agencies and faculties, and still are by some. Researchers are self-driven to inquire. They are controlled by their habits, the rules of funding, and their disciplines. Such forces control whether or not they will report their use of qualitative methods. All researchers depend on qualitative thinking, as set forth in these words by psychometrician Robert Mislevy:

> All the quantitative models that we talk about are overlaid over some substantive model that concerns the concepts, the entities, the relationships, and the events that they are supposed to be about. They are the tools to help us understand patterns in these terms. [In Figure 1.1 is] a diagram that sometimes we use in our classes to talk about this. (Mislevy, Moss, and Gee, 2008, p. 282)

Whether we are looking at the real world through quantitative or qualitative eyes, we reconceive the world in terms of the concepts and relationships of our experience. There are times when each researcher is going to be interpretive, holistic, naturalistic, and uninterested in cause, and at those times, by definition, he or she will be a qualitative researcher (see Glossary). But some of us, valuing the understandings potentially to be reached through qualitative study, will be qualitative inquirers most of the time.

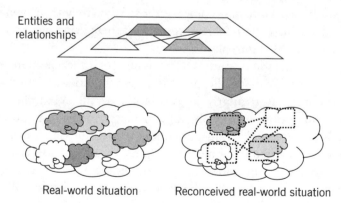

Entities and relationships

Real-world situation   Reconceived real-world situation

FIGURE 1.1. Illustration of general knowledge. *Source*: Mislevy et al., 2008. Copyright by Routledge. Reprinted by permission.

1.9. ESSENCE OF THE QUALITATIVE APPROACH

It is common for people to suppose that qualitative research is marked by rich description of personal action and complex environment, and it is, but the qualitative approach is equally distinguished, as I have claimed earlier in this chapter, for the integrity of its thinking. There is no one way of qualitative thinking, but a grand collection of ways: It is interpretive, experience based, situational, and personalistic. Each researcher will do it differently, but almost all of them will work hard at interpretation. They will try to convey some of the story in experiential terms. They will show the complexity of the background, and they will treat individuals as unique, yet in ways similar to other individuals.

Galileo did not reveal all those characteristics in his astronomical journals, but his thinking emphasized that even the most regular events, the movement of earth and stars, were available for reinterpretation. He relied upon his own experience, and he respected contexts. He did not study human beings formally, so he did not emphasize the personalistic side of qualitative research.

Qualitative research has moved social research away from an emphasis on cause-and-effect explanation and toward personal interpretation. Qualitative inquiry is distinguished by its emphasis on holistic treatment of phenomena (Silverman, 2000). I have remarked already on the epistemology of qualitative researchers as existential (nondeterministic) and constructivist. These two views are correlated with an expectation that phenomena are intricately related to many coincidental actions and that understanding them requires a wide sweep of contexts: temporal and spatial, historical, political, economic, cultural, social, personal.

Thus the case, the activity, the event, the thing is seen as unique as well as common. Understanding the case requires an understanding of other cases, things, and events but also an emphasis on its uniqueness. Such uniqueness is established not particularly by comparing it on a number of variables (there may be few ways in which this case differs from the norm), but the collection of features and the sequence of happenings are seen by people close at hand as (in several ways) unprecedented, a critical uniqueness. Readers can be drawn easily to this sense of uniqueness when we provide experiential accounts.

For all the intrusion into habitats and personal affairs, most qualitative researchers are noninterventionists: (can you forgive this stereotype?) They shy away from instigating an activity to study the thing. Most qualitative researchers try not to draw attention to themselves or their style of work. Other than positioning themselves, they avoid creating situations "to test their hypotheses." They try to observe the ordinary, and they try to observe it long enough to comprehend what, for this thing, "ordinary" means. For them, naturalistic observation has been their primary medium of acquaintance. When they cannot see for themselves, they ask others who have seen. When there are formal records kept, they search for the documents. But they favor a personal capture of the experience, so they can interpret it, recognize its contexts, puzzle the many meanings even while still there, and pass along an experiential, naturalistic account so that readers can participate in some of the same reflection. (Of course, qualitative researchers differ one from the other.)

In Box 1.3 we have a vignette written from an hour's visit to a university classroom in Mexico City. After you have read it, please contemplate again the essence of the qualitative approach. This account need not have been written so informally, but it was intended to capture the experience of being there. Description of the people, the place, the passing of time, were included to make it experiential, situational, and personalistic. Nothing is said as to the purpose for the observation, the use that might be made of it. Surely, on arrival, the observer had some question, some curiosity, and left with further questions. It doesn't become qualitative research until this kind of description is fitted to a research question. What might it be here? The quest for learning? The idiosyncrasies of teaching? The appetite for revolution? You are the interpreter.

You might find such a vignette in a qualitative research report. It emphasizes personal experience, the particular situation, and knowledge of the classroom as a teacher might know it. The data are there for microanalysis and interpretation. I tried to make a diagram to show the main concepts of this chapter, particularly the ties of qualitative research to individual experience, particularistic and situational learning, professional knowledge, and microanalysis. The best I managed to do is Figure 1.2, a figure not easy to understand. Perhaps you could make a better graphic to show it. I wanted to show those strong ties, but also that qualitative inquiry has ties with scientific and collective knowledge, with generalization, and with macroanalysis. Heavy and light lines connecting the circles are supposed to distinguish between the strong and weaker ties. Qualitative and quantitative inquiry have important differences, but, as the whirligig indicates, they also have lots of overlap and connections.

BOX 1.3. Class Notes, October 23, Mexico City

The temperature will climb into the 70s today, but now it is chilly in this white tile and terrazzo classroom. Eleven students (of 29 still on the roster) are here, each in a jacket or sweater. No doubt it was cooler when they left home. The instructor, Señor Pretelin, reminds them of the topic, the origins of capitalism, and selects a question for which they have prepared answers. An answer from the back row is ventured. Two more students arrive. It is ten past the hour. Now four more. Sr. Pretelin undertakes correction of the answer but asks for still more of an answer. His style is casual. He draws long on a cigarette. His audience is alert. Marx is a presence, spoken in name, and looming from the cover of the textbook. Two books only are in sight. Several students have photocopies of the chapter assigned. The chalkboard remains filled with last class's logic symbols, now unnoticed. Some students read through their answers; most concentrate on what Pretelin says about answers that are offered. The first answers had been volunteered by males, now one from a female. The instructor draws her out, more of her idea, then improves upon the explanation himself.

The coolness of the space is warmed by the exchanges. Outside a power mower sputters, struggling with a thickness of grass for which it probably was not designed. It is 20 past the hour. Another student arrives. Most are around 20, all have black hair. These are incoming freshmen in the social studies and humanities program, enrolled in a sociology course on political doctrines. Still another arrives. She pushes the door closed and jams it with a chair to thwart the breeze from the squared-out plaza. Sr. Pretelin is expanding an answer at length. He then turns to another question, lights another cigarette while awaiting a volunteer. Again he asks for improvement, gets a couple of tries, then answers the question to his satisfaction. Another question. He patiently awaits student initiative. The students appear to think or read to themselves what they had written earlier.

The haze of Mexico City shrouds the city center several miles to the southeast. Yesterday's downpour did not long cleanse the sky. Quiet again while awaiting a volunteer. The first young woman offers her answer. She is the only female of the seven or so students who have ventured forth. Heads nod to her reference to the campesinos [farm laborers]. If capitalistic advocacy exists in this classroom, it does not speak out. A half hour has passed. The recital continues. Only a few students are correcting their notes (or creating them belatedly), most try

(cont.)

BOX 1.3. *(cont.)*

to read or listen. Minds are mobilized, not idling. Finally a small wedge of humor.

The air may relax a bit. Four observers are dispersed about the room, little noticed even as they write. The instructor maintains his task, not ever stopping to take roll. Pretelin is a slight man, perhaps 40. He wears a smart jacket, a dark shirt buttoned high, a gold neck chain. His fingers are long and expressive. For several minutes, the dragging of heavy objects outside the room interferes. For a last time the students are sent to their answers, even asked to look further. Few have books. Then the students are invited to pose questions. The exchange becomes more good-natured but business-like still. The engagement goes on, minds "full on," provoked sociably, heads nodding agreement. More immediate campesinos, now drawn 17 million strong to the streets below, make the noises of the city. A poster admonishes: "Adman. Vota. Platestda." Near the door the graffiti begins, "La ignorancia mata. . . . " The hour draws to a close, a final cigarette, a summary, a warm smile.

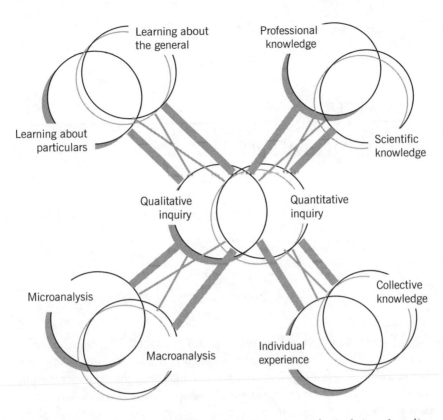

FIGURE 1.2. A whirligig of strong and weaker epistemological ties of qualitative Inquiry.

CHAPTER 2

Interpretation
The Person as Instrument

Research is not a machine to grind out facts. The main machine in all research is a human researcher. Or a team of humans. In qualitative research, the humans have a lot to do, planning the study, arranging for situations to observe, interviewing people, examining records, putting patches of ideas together, writing reports. When you think about using instruments in research, you need to include humans as some of the main instruments.

Humans are the researchers. Humans are being studied. Humans are the interpreters, among them the readers of our reports.

2.1. INTERPRETIVE RESEARCH

Qualitative research is sometimes defined as *interpretive research*. All research requires interpretations, and, in fact, human behavior requires interpretation minute by minute. But interpretive research is investigation that relies heavily on observers defining and redefining the meanings of what they see and hear. If no one is hurt, something like a car crash may mean pretty much the same to people—just crush and crumple—but as they think about it, some see the crash as negligence, some as fate, and some as need for stricter laws. Their interpretations are not only what they think after they have stopped to think about it but are part of the seeing. The perceptions we have of objects and events and relationships are simultaneously interpretive. They get continuing reinterpretation. Qualitative research draws heavily on interpreting by researchers—and also on interpreting by the people they study and by the readers of the research reports.

As you know, interpretations can be faulty. Part of learning how to do qualitative research is learning how to minimize the flaws in our observations and assertions. We will "triangulate" our data in order to increase confidence that we have correctly interpreted how things work. Sometimes our views are faulty because they are too simplistic. A car crash has multiple causes. So does a scolding. How things work can be more complicated than they seem at first. Triangulation will help us recognize that things need more explanation than we at first thought.

Here's an example. Suppose you apply for a fellowship. You wonder how other applicants, your competitors, are making their applications appealing. You ask some people what they think and conclude that the winning applications will be those portraying a "well-rounded personality." There, you did a tiny qualitative study, asking a complex question and making an interpretation. Your interpretation of those data may have been well reasoned but, for your purpose, faulty. Too little evidence. It could be that these judges are giving highest ratings to applicants not well rounded but who have concentrated on a very few unusual activities (fruit tree grafting and debate competition, as examples). Had you struggled harder, had you triangulated your finding, perhaps by asking previous winners and looking on the web for the rationale of the competition, you might have reached a better interpretation. But that is common sense, you say. Yes, qualitative research is disciplined common sense.

Furthermore, the interpretations of qualitative research give emphasis to human values and experiences. Norman Denzin, an advocate of interpretive interactionism (a form of qualitative research) has said:

> Interpretive interactionism attempts to make the meanings that circulate in the world of lived experience accessible to the reader. It endeavors to capture and represent the voices, emotions, and actions of those studied. The focus of interpretive research is on those life experiences that radically alter and shape the meanings persons give to themselves and their experiences. (2001, p. 1)

So that is one way of doing qualitative research: finding the meanings of personally transformative experience. Figuring out the "Wow!" in a lifetime.

But other qualitative researchers are more intent on understanding ordinary behavior, such as walking a child to kindergarten or repairing a tire. It usually is not this walking thing or repairing thing itself but what it tells of family protection or self-reliance. Many anthropologists urge researchers to study not what is extraordinary but what is common. Here, again, is contention between social science's interest in the generalizable and predictable and the social action and professional service interest in the unique case, the situational. Both can be served by qualitative research.

Denzin (2001) also spoke of "critical" interpretive study, meaning "important," of course, but also meaning "interpreting things in terms of particular value commitments" (sometimes ideological, such as feminist or Christian or social justice beliefs) for the purpose of contributing to improvement of the human condition. Being a social activist or evangelist can be part of research, or it can be a role assumed alongside research, kept separate. The researcher has a choice. Researchers have so many choices, if their jobs permit it. Sometimes those choices are more or less decided for them. The choices of view have long been a part of research.

These are choices for each researcher. Interpretive interactionism is not the only way of doing qualitative research, not even a very common way. Opponents to any particular social action or to reform broadly can also do qualitative research. The methods are there for anyone to use, but it is common to find the majority of qualitative researchers inclined to interpret the way things work more along the lines of left-wing politics than right-wing politics. That's the way people have been lining up, but it's not part of the definition.

There is no clear border between common sense interpretation, reform-minded interpretation, and research interpretation. Research interpretation will usually be deliberated, abstract, and literary. When the procedures for deliberation are formalized, laid out step by step, we might capitalize it as Interpretive Research to distinguish it from daily thinking and advocacy. A good qualitative research project will deal deeply with a few of the complexities of human experience. It will draw upon the best thinking, the best writing of people, past and present; thus it is literary. For that reason we review the research literature. But perhaps the most distinctive feature of qualitative research is that it is interpretive, a struggle with meanings.

2.2. MICROINTERPRETATION AND MACROINTERPRETATION

A researcher's struggle with meanings occurs in many places and takes many forms, but one important distinction among interpretations is between those small and personally oriented and those large and societially oriented. It also is situational thinking versus universal thinking. In Section 1.3 we made the distinction between macroresearch and microresearch. Now we make a similar distinction between microinterpretation and macrointerpretation. How things generally work is a macrointerpretation. How a particular thing works in a particular situation is a microinterpretation. Both use qualitative research, but most of the time qualitative research results in microinterpretation.

Microinterpretation is giving meaning in terms of what an individual person can experience, such as climbing a particular tree, or listening to the opening movement of a concerto while driving home, or becoming acquainted with the cooking course your friend took. You might think of it as a single instance, something like a single "measurement," however complicated, in the form of human experience. If you were to analyze the dialogue between two marines, we could call the analysis *microanalysis*, and the meanings that you give to their expressions would be microinterpretation. Lots of good qualitative research relies on microinterpretation.[1]

Macrointerpretation is making meaning in terms of what large groups of people (or machines or other bodies) do, such as choosing a president, preparing for college, or nursing infants. Individuals, of course, experience voting, preparing for college, and nursing babies, but when we think of that experience over great numbers of people, it is generalized, getting a special kind of interpretation. It creates a different kind of knowledge. Here in the United States we conceptualize blue states and red states, states having majorities of Democratic and Republican voting. We conceptualize general increases in tuition. We think not so much of the extraordinary closeness of a mother and nursing infant

---

[1]In his *Dictionary of Terms*, Thomas Schwandt (1997) defines a method called microethnography as

> a particular type of qualitative inquiry specifically concerned with exhaustive, fine-grained examination of either a very small unit within an organization, group or culture (e.g., a particular classroom in a school); a specific activity within an organizational unit (e.g., how physicians communicate with elderly patients in an emergency room); or ordinary everyday conversation. (p. 94)

but of a generalization such as the onset of lactose intolerance. We may call the study of these experiences across many instances "macroanalysis" and the interpretation of the observations "macrointerpretation."

It is easy to think of these two, the micro and the macro, as shading into each other, from small numbers of experiences to large, but it is difficult to get to general knowledge from particular knowledge, no matter the number of people involved. Patterns of immigration are not easy to learn by studying individual immigrants. Is there gradual shading or a discrete change from general knowledge to particular knowledge? And from particular to general? Something to think about.

In this book we are most interested in research on instances, particulars, cases, narratives, situations, and episodes—on how individual things work. Qualitative research primarily calls for microanalysis and microinterpretation. In the following example from the 1970s, the researcher presents what happened in one school being newly equipped for teaching and learning, including the provision of chairs. The episode called for microinterpretation, but the researcher, David Hamilton, was also intent upon generalization, upon macrointerpretation. He wanted the reader to think about the general policy of equipping schools and how it relates to the methods of teaching in those classrooms.

To tell his story, Hamilton (no date) alluded to the role of researcher as detective, teasing out assumptions, uncovering reasons for practice, and delving into myths and dogma. The portion quoted in Box 2.1 was abstracted from his in-depth study of a Scottish open-plan school.[2] He presents "the case of the missing chairs." In the process he uncovers a number of relationships, patches, microinterpretations, and macrointerpretations.

We examine this report as an example of microanalysis of primary school teaching, but the author's interpretations as to school policy and empathy for teachers' beliefs put macroanalysis out in front. The report also should help us think about the difficulty of condensing the experience of the researcher on-site to the few words of a report.

(text resumes on p. 46)

---

[2]The reading is long, but it is a good place in this book to think of research as its embodiment in a report. Several ideas (such as particularization, interpretation, subjectivity, and causality) expressed on earlier pages are to be found in this report. The reading should help clarify the distinction between micro- and macrointerpretation. But to me, your experience in reading Hamilton's report is more important than its content. Understanding how things work is a matter of experience.

BOX 2.1. The Case of the Missing Chairs

DAVID HAMILTON, *Scottish Council for Research in Education*

There is a school of thought in primary education that argues that there is no need to provide every child with a seat or a work surface. Support for this idea comes from various sources. New schools find the concept financially acceptable since it releases money from an otherwise fixed grant for the purchase of specialist furnishings such as display screens, storage units and mobile trolleys. Architects endorse the idea since the resultant increase in free space enables them to create more flexible designs. And finally, educationalists lend their weight to the scheme since it visibly undermines a long tradition of simultaneous class (i.e., whole group) teaching.

The force of these economic, architectural and educational arguments has been considerable. According to one recent English review: "new purpose-built open plan schools rarely contain seating accommodation for more than about seventy percent of the children at any one time." Not all practitioners, however, have found this innovation equally acceptable. Hence, like many other elements in the modern primary school, chairs and tables have become the object of prolonged and often emotive debate. Superficially, the arguments and counter-arguments are about the allocation of financial resources and the utilisation of available space. At a deeper level, however, they also interact with more fundamental concerns about the theory and practice of primary education. In short, discussions about tables and chairs are also debates about methods and curricula.

The first part of this article explores the origins and assumptions of these debates. The second part relates their logic to the experience of a case study school. Throughout, two questions are considered:

1. What are the shifts in educational thinking that have given rise to these discussions?
2. How do these shifts relate to a reduced provision of chairs?

The standard answer to these questions is that a lowered requirement of chairs follows automatically from a weaker emphasis upon class and jotter-based teaching. The experience of the case study school (and the argument of this essay) suggests that the case for this innovation is weak and inconclusive.

(cont.)

BOX 2.1. *(cont.)*

CHAIRS: A VANISHING RESOURCE?

At some point in the late 1960s (or so it appears) the idea began to circulate that a primary school could be efficiently furnished with less than one hundred per cent seating. The source of this notion is as yet obscure. The fact that there are no references to it in either the Plowden Report (1967) or the Scottish Education Department "Primary Memorandum" (1965) suggests that it may have been a grass-roots or even an imported (American?) idea.

The rationale for limiting the number of chairs in a school derives from three assumptions:

1. That the basic unit of teaching should be the individual child rather than the whole group.
2. That it is possible to organise work programmes whereby children can be employed on different activities.
3. That not all learning activities require a chair.

There are two problems with this rationale. First, none of these assumptions specifically requires that the provision of seats should be fixed at less than one hundred percent. In fact, it would be possible for a teacher to accept all three ideas and still legitimately demand a full complement of chairs. This would follow, for example, if she added a fourth assumption: that children should be free to choose their own sequence through the various activities of their work programme. Indeed, if a teacher considered this last assumption to be the most important, then it would definitely rule out a reduced provision of chairs. The freedom of individual choice would, by necessity, include the freedom for every child to choose a seated activity. Thus, to restrict the number of chairs in a school is automatically to limit the number of curriculum options open to teachers and pupils. Certainly, an increase of chairs may also produce a shortage of space; but this is not an equivalent problem. Space can be created more easily than extra seating.

The second problem surrounds the levels of seating that are usually considered as realistic (i.e., sixty to seventy percent). The derivation of these figures is as obscure as the origins of the initial idea. It is sometimes stated that a sixty-six percent (i.e., two-thirds) seating level fits easily where classes are subdivided into three groups. In such cases the expectation is that two thirds of the class group will need chairs

(cont.)

BOX 2.1. *(cont.)*

whereas one third will be working at non-seated activities or out of the class area. On balance this explanation is inadequate. It does not justify the choice of three groups or indicate how a policy of group squares with the assumption that the individual child should be the basic teaching unit. (By the same token it would be just as reasonable to divide the class into four groups and have a seating level seventy-five or even fifty percent.)

Given the educational weakness of the foregoing argument, an alternative source for the quoted figures is that they derive from the application of a standard architectural formula. By this means a school's optimum seating requirements are calculated in the same manner as the size of playground and staffroom. Nevertheless, these requirements cannot be predicted unambiguously. They also depend on the kind of educational policy followed by a school. An optimum figure in one situation may be totally inappropriate in another.

ACCIDENTAL DISSEMINATION?

The rather hybrid nature of these ideas about seating levels suggests that they may have come into being for no other purpose than to focus attention on out-of-date classroom procedures. That is, they were formulated primarily to draw attention to the shortcomings of educational practice not as a model for changing it.

If this last explanation is in fact correct, then the initial adoption of reduced seating levels may have been accidental—the reluctant or ill-informed act of a financially hard-pressed adviser administrator. Whatever their origins, the rapid widespread dissemination of these ideas was almost certainly attributable to concerned pressure of administrators, college lecturers and architects: three powerful groups in primary education. Although acting for different reasons—expediency, conviction or functional utility—their combined advocacy has been considerable.

AT SCHOOL LEVEL

In the early 1970s teachers from the case study school attended a local college of education for courses leading to the Froebel (early education) certificate. During those years, they first encountered the idea that a

(cont.)

BOX 2.1. *(cont.)*

primary school class might be organised around less than one hundred per cent seating. At that time, however, the issue was of academic rather than practical concern, a matter for staffroom discussion rather than school-wide decision.

In 1973 the situation changed. The plans for the new lower primary building had reached the stage where a seating level had to be decided. Consensus among the staff was difficult to achieve since individual members reacted differently to the idea that seating levels might be reduced below one chair per child. Basically, three viewpoints were expressed. One (small) group of teachers were prepared to put their beliefs to the test and try out the idea. A second group (probably the majority) accepted the general notion of a reduced provision but felt that their own situation constituted a special case. For example, one teacher argued that she preferred to teach writing by means of class lessons. A third group of teachers were less easily converted. They felt reluctant to abandon either the principle or the practice of providing a full complement of seats for their children. A characteristic feature of this last group was that they felt it was educationally important that each child should have their "own" chair.

To resolve this issue the headmaster of the school was asked to act as an arbitrator. By his decision the seating level was duly fixed at sixty percent. In principle this action closed the debate. In practice, however, the teachers were left with a possible alternative: if the designated seating level proved inadequate, it could still be topped up with infant-sized furniture left over from the old buildings. The flexibility of this arrangement became apparent when some of the ordered furniture failed to arrive in time for the opening of the new building. The old tables and chairs were immediately pressed into service and, in a complete reversal of the original intention, were "topped up" by the new furniture as it arrived. Eventually, a surplus of chairs was created—which meant that each teacher could operate their own seating policy. Some chose the figure of sixty percent while others retained at least one chair for each child.

This arrangement did not last for very long. Within a term all the teachers had built up their seating levels to at least one hundred percent. The topping up, however, did not herald a return to class teaching. Quite the reverse: it marked a recognition that an adequate supply

(cont.)

BOX 2.1. *(cont.)*

of chairs was necessary to the individualised and balanced curriculum that the case study teachers were trying to implement. Thus, despite a certain sense of public failure among the teachers who tried to work with a reduced provision, the intervening experience had taught them a great deal about the relationship between teaching methods and seating requirements.

AT CLASSROOM LEVEL

The teachers who found themselves unable to operate with a reduction in chairs reported the following experiences. In the first instance they all found it impossible to avoid times when their entire teaching group was sitting on chairs. Sometimes this arose through the teacher's own decision; at other times it arose through the actions of the children. Although the frequency of these occasions was rare and their duration short-lived, the teachers regarded them as an essential part of their work. In so far as these experiences served educational purposes that could not be achieved in any other way, the teachers were unwilling to abandon them for the sake of a handful of chairs.

A second experience related to the use of chairs as a moveable resource. The teachers conceded that it might be possible to use less than one hundred percent chairs for much of the school day but had found that this usually required a certain proportion of chairs to be moved constantly from place to place. This occurred, for example, when a group of children wanted to set up a "school" in the "shop," or a "hairdressing salon" in the home base. The teachers not only felt that the movement of chairs created avoidable disruption but also that the associated shortage of chairs inhibited their pupil's choice of activity.

A third observation (made by the teachers of younger children) was that a limited supply of chairs could interfere with the educational principle that certain well-used areas or activities (e.g., milk, sewing, reading) should have a fixed allocation of chairs. The justification for this policy was that the presence of chairs could help children to perform activities that might otherwise be too difficult. It was also argued in favour of such a policy that it helped to prevent certain practical problems (e.g., spillage of milk, loss of sewing needles, damage of books). In

(cont.)

BOX 2.1. *(cont.)*

these instances the combined weight of the educational and administrative advantages was sufficient to convince the teachers of the need for extra chairs.

Finally, all the teachers reported that they were unwilling to allow children to write while standing at a work surface or lying on the floor. The notion that children should be allowed to write in these positions has been one of the outcomes of the chairs debate. Without exception, the case study teachers reacted unfavourably to the idea. Like the erstwhile master of St. Andrew's Grammar School, they felt that children who are learning to write should be encouraged to use a suitable surface and a comfortable chair.

CONCLUSION

This article examines a rather curious discrepancy between theory and practice. It focuses on a school of thought which holds that a modern primary school can be adequately equipped with less than one chair per child. Overall, it questions the practice whereby chairs are shared rather than a guaranteed resource. In effect, this means that chairs are downgraded to the same status as painting easels, water tanks and sand trays. As a result, special rules are needed to regulate the pupils' access to them. In turn, these rules have an impact on the type of methods and curricula which can be used by teachers.

It may be expedient to improve the provision of the painting easels at the expense of chairs. But, in the process, there is surely no need to make an educational virtue out of an economic necessity.

Source: Hamilton (no date). Reprinted with permission from the Scottish Council for Research in Education.

2.3. EMPATHY

As expressed in Box 1.2, characteristic 4, qualitative research is special in its personalistic orientation, relying on empathy with the humans and enterprises studied for understanding how things work. A dictionary will say that to empathize is to look at things closely, becoming sensitive to, even vicariously experiencing, the feelings, thoughts, and happenings.

Empathy is different from sympathy, which is a feeling of personal closeness, endearment, and solace, a feeling of emotional accord. With empathy—which is a matter of perception more than emotion—it is easier, I think, to work for negotiation and problem solving. It is unlikely that empathy and sympathy will exist completely separately, but most qualitative researchers try to be empathic, less driven by sympathy. Empathy is a part of qualitative research, but, to be sure, the writings of some researchers will reflect empathy more than those of others.

In her 1995 book, *Medicine and the Family: A Feminist Perspective*, Lucy Candib spoke of qualitative research as "connected knowing." Connected knowing is the embodiment of empathy, using personal experiences and relationships to inquire how others see how things work. It relies on a studied perception of situations in context, thus working toward credibility and esteem.

One of the reminders of empathic inquiry is that the individual human is a complex person, similar in many ways to others but unique in personality and life situation. In their efforts to understand how social things work, most qualitative researchers treat each human being and the collective of all human beings as beyond full understanding. They do not aspire to an eventual full understanding, expecting that the lives of people will become ever more complex even as we reach any new insight. We study human affairs not expecting to pin down their fundamental nature, for that knowledge is well beyond the construction of what we can know.

Anthropologist Ivan Brady (2006) wrote:

> Is there some common ground that can be apprehended through the trowels, brushes, and screens of the senses that will give us a realistic impression of life in ancient places and thereby address the concerns of our environmental critics? We are one species, one subspecies in biological form, embodied more or less the same everywhere, and as conscious beings we need to know (or think we know) where we are before we are able to choose definitive courses of action. The comparative framework provided by that posture gives us access to other humans through sympathy and empathy, that is, by tapping in "fellow feeling" with speculation and imagination at work, both of which are essential parts of the interpretive equation. (p. 982)

To gain access to humans, to understand their stories, Brady challenges us to use both sympathy and empathy. Researchers will decide for themselves how sympathetic to be. A qualitative researcher has no choice but to be empathic.

2.4. THICK DESCRIPTION AND *VERSTEHEN*

Researchers base their interpretations of how things work on understanding, sometimes by understanding measurements and models. Qualitative researchers reach many (perhaps most) of their interpretations instead through experiential understanding. It may be understanding from their own personal experience or from the recollections and artifacts of the personal experience of others. They sometimes refer to experiential understanding as *verstehen*.

The German word for personal understanding, *verstehen* (vair stay' en), may come to be one of the most important words for you as a qualitative researcher. Persuasively, philosopher William Dilthey argued that knowledge in the human sciences is greatly different from that in the physical sciences, the second being impersonal explanations of how things work, the first being what humans think and feel as to how things work. It was not that humans draw conclusions with little evidence, which is often true, but that, no matter how shy or subdued they are, they understand events as somehow a participant in them. *Verstehen* is an experiential understanding of action and context.

Gabriel García Márquez wrote *One Hundred Years of Solitude* about the happenings in the Arcadio Buendía family across a century. In qualitative research we write about what actually happened, not about fiction, but we write also about what people say they experience. There is more than a pinch of fiction in what people say. And in what we research writers say as well.

We will not plunge into how we write reports until much later in the book. This chapter is on interpretation. But the interpretations we write are shaped greatly by what we have experienced. Writing is not a printer printing, not just putting on paper what was stored in memory. Research writing is rich with interpretation. And interpretation is shaped by a need to get things written. Columnist James Reston said, "How do I know what I think until I read what I write." Writing is a form of thinking.

To assist our readers' understanding we describe the action, the dialogue, the people, their contexts, and the passage of time. We make rich descriptions. We try to make it easy for them to incorporate our descriptions into their own experience. We know they will make different interpretations, because they have their own experience to go on too. And their experience becomes more complex as they experience vicariously the action we describe.

Toward the end of *One Hundred Years of Solitude*, García Márquez (1970)[3] described how Úrsula, at age 100, dealt with her blindness, fixing on the routines of others, learning to time the heating of milk, threading a needle. García Márquez pondered the meanings of old age and blindness, but he did not make connections with the vast research on those topics or any scholarly study of family interdependency. He was not writing a social science research paper. His description is rich, but not what we have come to call *thick description*.

Thick description is a concept offered by anthropologist Clifford Geertz, one of the great persons of qualitative research. In 1993 he wrote a monograph, *Thick Description, Toward an Interpretive Theory of Culture*. Notice the emphasis on interpretation, not asking just for detailed description, but asking for thinking about theory. His aim was to see the thing as part of sociocultural science. We might consider what does it mean for Úrsula to be 100 years old? Limited vision? Limited access? Dependency? A description is rich if it provides abundant, interconnected details, and possibly cultural complexity, but it becomes *thick* description if it offers direct connection to cultural theory and scientific knowledge.

Geertz urged that qualitative researchers describe the situation well, have empathic understanding, and compare present interpretations with those in the research literature. He urged us to examine closely what is happening in front of us so that we can ponder meanings deeply and offer pertinent vicarious experiences to our readers. But especially he urged us to question theory. Here is an example of thick description that I borrow from Rob Walker (1978) about a science teacher in a progressive high school over 30 years ago.

[Daniel] feels it is important to approach the experience of materials through aesthetics rather than explanation. He stresses the ordinariness of

---

[3] You could look it up. The quotation came from the outset of a chapter beginning with the words, "In the bewilderment of her last years, Úrsula . . ." In my 383-page copy, it is on page 230. The author did not number the chapters.

many of the things he uses: starch, soap bubbles, milk cartons. "You've got to get teachers confident enough to play with materials," he says, "because they have got to be confident enough to get the materials into the hands of the students, and to tolerate them playing around with them." . . .

Around the room are some samples of the work that is going on in Daniel's courses. A tray of starch has dried out to leave characteristic crack lines. ("It looks random at first sight, but there are some interesting patterns. Notice how the lines are mostly perpendicular to one another.") In a plastic bucket is a water wheel made out of milk cartons. When the wheel turns, it winds up a winch. ("First of all you just play with it. Then you ask, 'Does it go further if you tip a cup of sand in slow or fast? Do two cups wind it twice as far as one cup?' Once you get started there's no end to what you can do.")

[For him] the problem with most teacher education courses, and with in-service courses, lies in the implicit view they have of the teacher. "Most of the teacher institutes I have had anything to do with," Daniel says, "have been concerned to promote or to implement some already worked-out curriculum. It is very rare for the people who are running them to find out where the teacher is, and start from there" (pp. 11–33).

Walker saw the theoretical implication of Daniel's words for project-method teaching, for teacher education, and for common standards.

In your own fieldwork interpretations, you may sometimes make thick description a high priority. But sometimes seeking thick description will distract your interpreting a particular experience. When should your interpretation move from the particular to the general? Thick description will tell of the particular but pushes us toward thinking about generalizations. We ask and we watch, expecting people's words and actions to reveal their engagement in situations. To a degree they are fiction, but as research we hold them dear because, after we see them again and again, they yield *verstehen,* understandings of how things work for those people.

2.5. CONTEXT AND SITUATION

Context and situation are background. They are important to the story, but they are not what the research is about. Our interpretations depend on good understanding of surrounding conditions, the context and situation. The research is about an activity or group or relationship. This is the content of the research but not the context. The content is foreground; the context is background.

Suppose you are studying Madeleine. You aren't studying her just because she will make an interesting story. You study her because you want to understand her better. Your research question will tell what about Madeleine makes her interesting to study. The context will be some of the circumstances most helpful for understanding her. Actually, there are several contexts—for example, her family context, her school context, and her religious context. That doesn't mean how she interacts with her family, school, and church but what we should try to understand about her family, school, and church as background to her actions.

Suppose you are next going to study your own group (classroom, caseload, department). You might call it action research or self-study. You may be facing a particular problem, such as lack of communication or your reputation. Or one of the group is not fitting in very well. You need to understand the situation better. What are the surrounding conditions? What are the priorities? What are the problems? How are those priorities and problems seen differently? You know some of the answers, but you need to know more. It could be that there is more historical, political, economic, or aesthetic background than you now know. Raising questions about contexts may help you increase your understanding. Problem solving sometimes needs to wait for better understanding.

In Chapter 8 you will read about the bubble gum experiment. There were several important contexts. It was a school with a strong emphasis on teacher continuing education, particularly in art and mathematics. The school was in a poor neighborhood with parents strongly supporting the school. It was a time of national emphasis on improving test scores, more than on having experiences such as doing experiments. In the total report, these contexts were developed further than in the excerpt you will read. Some important contexts come to the researcher's mind by thinking of the areas of human study: psychology, culture, history, economics, and politics. For the bubble gum experiment,[4] there also was an ethical context. The teacher, Miss Grogan, stopped the experiment to find out who was guilty of stealing the bubble gum. The context was important, as in this paragraph:

---

[4]More on the bubble gum experiment appears in Section 8.2.

> This more or less unconscious choice between academic learning opportunity and social ethics opportunity was not uncommon in elementary schools generally but was seldom discussed. It was the teacher's sense of propriety that decided, and the choice made by Grogan would be supported regularly by the other teachers and parents. When asked about it, a number of children in this District's schools also had expressed support for maintaining decorum and punishing misbehavior, even at the cost of good learning activities. (Stake, 2000, p. 24)

The researcher felt it useful in helping the reader understand Grogan's teaching to interrupt the story to speak of the high priority on ethical decorum in that classroom. The reader's understanding of what happened in that mathematics class probably is influenced by the teacher's efforts to punish the thief and, more broadly, by the ethical context.

"Context" tends to be thought of as rather stable, something that does not change much from day to day. "Situation" is a more immediate background, the things that are going on right now behind the main activities of study. Often, there will be no clear boundaries between what is foreground and what is background; they blend into each other. The episode of the bubble gum experiment (this patch) was more understandable because it occurred at the end of the school year, after end-of-year tests, when strict emphasis on curriculum guidelines diminishes. That was part of the situation in which we will find Grogan's students experimenting with bubble gum.

Situations are extra important for qualitative research. The theorists invented the word "situationality," referring to the attention given to particular places, times, social backgrounds, communication styles, and other backgrounds for the activities and relationships being studied. The situation provides part of the meaning for qualitative phenomena.

Qualitative research differs from much quantitative research by giving careful study to contexts. A few context variables are included in many quantitative studies, but most others are treated as unimportant, not contributing to grand understanding of the main effects. Some quantitative studies may look at parents' hopes for a "return to normality" of children with autism. Qualitative studies may also look at parents' hopes for a return to normality, looking at a relatively few cases, paying attention to the presence of siblings, age of parents, their general knowledge of the disability, religious affiliation, the perspectives of teachers, medical resources, community services for those with disability, the mainstreaming movement, and other background characteristics. Quantitative studies could include measurements of these background variables, and some do. But there is an important difference. Qualitative researchers expect to devote much of their interpretation to context and situation. It is part of their sense of how things work. Quantitative researchers concentrate on the differences, such as age of parents, that can be counted as being part of the explanation of parental hope across the population of families of children with autism. They treat fewer influences at a time. It is part of their sense of how things work.

All this does not mean that a study cannot have parts that are quantitative and parts that are qualitative. And that does not mean that you need to decide which you are more loyal to.

Contexts are important. It would not surprise me if some qualitative researchers would include in their reports a "table of contexts" as well as a table of contents.

2.6. SKEPTICISM

People of all personalities should be involved in qualitative research. It is not just a matter of equal opportunity; it is important to have data gathered by people with different psychological dispositions. Each will add something different to the understanding of a research question. Understanding shifts with the accomplishments of large numbers of people, even though a few may be in special ways more expert than the rest. And the accomplishments of the research community are measured in the accomplishments of all who study human processes.

But one personal characteristic needed at least some of the time by almost all researchers is skepticism. Much of the time, researchers need to be dissatisfied with what they know and with the evidence available. It should regularly be seen as inadequate. Available understanding and evidence will often have to suffice, because problems need to be acted upon. And waiting until later is seldom going to increase understanding and evidence substantially. We talk more about evidence in Chapter 7.

Cheer, faith, and trust are desirable in our fellow men and women, and we would not build good social services without those traits. But doubt is also a great virtue. Doubt that immobilizes can be hurtful, but doubt can be a protective shield. Doubt can cause digging toward better understanding.

You don't want your spouse, your parents, or your children to be compulsively skeptical. You do want your doctor, your mechanic, and your city council representative to be consistently skeptical. You want these caretakers to be persistently looking for what could be wrong.

And as you design your research, as you gather data, as you interpret what works, and as you explain to others what you are finding, you need a disposition to doubt. You need to suppose you are not getting the meaning straight and need to dig deeper. The general strategy qualitative researchers use for expressing doubt is called *triangulation*, something we work on in Chapter 7. By increasing care in gathering data and interpreting them, we increase assurance that we are on the right track and decrease tolerance for inaction.

Skepticism can lead to seeing complication and multiple realities, but many people do not want to hear about complexity, and prefer to think that "the thing" is simple.

Doubts

The more you doubt the issue
The less you'll be deceived.
With questioning of the mission
From obligation you're relieved.
The longer we are skeptical,
More possibilities are conceived.
But however we speak our doubts,
Most simplicities stay believed.

Sometimes we need to be more skeptical than at other times. Right while gathering data from a person, it is best to try to understand and respect what is being said. It is best to treat that fact or story as an important perception. But, soon after, note should be taken as to what needs to be checked further. And both the small pictures and the big picture should several times be examined for clues to other meanings as to what makes things work.

2.7. EMPHASIS ON INTERPRETATION

Qualitative researchers such as Frederick Erickson, Yvonna Lincoln, and I rely heavily on direct interpretation of events and less on interpreted measurements. All research has a dependence on interpretation, but with standard quantitative designs, there is an effort to limit the role of personal interpretation during that period between the time the design is set and the time the data are collected. Standard qualitative designs call for the persons most responsible for interpretations to be in the field making observations and making interpretations iteratively.

In an outstanding summary of the nature of qualitative study, anthropologist Frederick Erickson (1986) claimed that the primary characteristic of qualitative research is the priority given to interpretation. He said that the findings are not just findings but "assertions." These assertions are the best-developed meanings we give to the most important things, including "how they work." Given up-close interaction of the researcher with persons in the field, given a constructivist orientation to knowledge, given the attention to participant intentionality and sense of self, however descriptive the report, the researcher ultimately comes to put forward a personal interpretation, an assertion. Erickson drew attention to the ethnographers' traditional emphasis on emic issues, those concerns and values recognized in the behavior and language of the people being studied. Thick description, alternative interpretations, and multiple realities are expected. Ongoing attention to complex meanings is much more difficult when the instruments of data gathering are objectively interpretable checklists as found in surveys. An ongoing, subjective, interpretive role of the researcher is common in the work of qualitative research.

Interpretation is an act of composition. The interpreter takes descriptions and makes them more complex, drawing upon a few conceptual relationships. He or she might take the term *work* and give it muscle, durability, remuneration, and self-respect. These can be some of the larger meanings of *work*. He or she might take an episode observed at the workplace and give it personality, history, tension, and implication. The best interpretations will be logical extensions of the simple description but also will include contemplative, speculative, even aesthetic extension. The reader would be deceived if allowed to think that these interpretations had been agreed upon, certified in some way. They are contributions of the researcher, written so as to make it clear they are personal interpretations. All people make interpretations. All research requires interpretations. Qualitative research relies heavily on interpretive perceptions throughout the planning, data gathering, analysis, and write-up of the study.

CHAPTER 3

Experiential Understanding
Most Qualitative Study Is Experiential

Qualitative inquiry and quantitative inquiry sometimes look like each other, but they are separated fundamentally (if not always cleanly) by their aims. It is an epistemological distinction, one based on a perception of knowledge that is personally "constructed" versus the one of knowledge as "discovery" of what the world is. Climbing trees is personally constructed knowledge. The function of tree roots is part of the world discovered in books or passed on by other authorities. The important distinction between qualitative and quantitative research is not based on the distinction between verbal description and numerical data. It is a difference between the study of personal knowledge versus the study of objective measurements.

A similar distinction exists between inquiry for making explanations versus inquiry for promoting understanding. This one was nicely developed by philosopher Georg Hendrik von Wright in his book *Explanation and Understanding* (1971). He conceded that explanations are intended to promote general understanding. He noted that understanding is often expressed in terms of explanation—but that the two are epistemologically different. Von Wright emphasized the difference between thinking of cause and effect (explanation) and the informal appreciation of experience (understanding).

It is a distinction a little bit like that between medicating the patient and nurturing the patient. Of course, we do both, but they are quite different, one much more personal than the other.

It is a distinction something like that between teacher-centered teaching and child-centered teaching. Preparing to teach in didactic fashion is different from arranging experiential opportunities for learners. Of course, many teachers do both.

Quantitative research tends to be an effort to improve the theoretical comprehension of the researchers, who in turn present it to their colleagues and students, and for practical application to diverse audiences. Qualitative research tends to be an effort to generate descriptions and situational interpretations of phenomena that the researcher can offer colleagues, students, and others for modifying their own understandings of phenomena (Stake and Trumbull, 1982).

A qualitative researcher tries to report a few, usually not a vast number of, situational experiences—not necessarily the most influential ones. He or she selects activities and contexts that provide opportunity to understand an interesting part of how the thing works. The range and completeness of experience studied is not as important as picking experiences that can be said to be insightful revelations, a good contribution to personal understanding.

3.1. THE PLACES OF HUMAN ACTIVITY

Whether full time or part time or only just for a while, you and I are "professional qualitative researchers." We are people who will make formal studies of social, educational, and similar things, usually programs and people. For the rest of our lives, we will be trying to improve our ability to understand how these things work.

Practitioners, program administrators, and many others also try to understand those programs and people. Usually they do it informally. We professional researchers boast, "Sometimes we can see the relationships more clearly, or find them in different forms, or find them more reliably." But we know, too, that people with special experience—people such as caregivers of all kinds, officials, even our children—can understand some things better than people with formal research training. Fortunate is the researcher who learns how to use the assistance of people with special experience!

We ask many questions: How good is the monitoring? How safe are the work spaces? How honest is the report? Is the library still a place for finding references? Was that a good experience for the people served? We try to answer such questions everywhere.

Most of the time we are not historians but examiners of the here and now. We study in the present tense, even though we may write it up in the past tense. We write of experience, experience in a place. The place influences how things work. The words of action researcher Stephen Kemmis (2007) can help us feel the importance of place (Box 3.1).

In particular places, we professional researchers look for better ways to discern how things are working (Brady, 2006). And we seek better ways to describe to others what we find. We look for ways to persuade the readers of our reports that our scores are pertinent and our interpretations trustworthy. What does that mean in your situation?

Around the world, today as in years past, much research has a strong political connection. Many people use research findings to promote their causes. Many people, including sponsors and agencies, do what they can to make the research design so that the findings will support their policies. The world of professional research is infused with politics. Does that mean that research reports cannot be trusted? Sometimes.

3.2. CRITERIAL AND EXPERIENTIAL DESCRIPTION

Evaluation theorists Daniel Stufflebeam and Anthony Shinkfield (2007) wrote about three ways professional researchers think about how things work: theories, models, and practices. That is right. Theirs is an emphasis on criterial thinking. After 40 years of working with educational researchers, I see another two fundamental ways researchers express themselves: criterially and experientially. Putting it criterially, I would say, "The weather was hot and humid." Putting it experientially, I would say, "His shirt was soon damp with sweat."

They say it differently, and they see it differently. Criterially, a researcher describes the world in scalar or dimensional language (using dimensions such as size, duration, and readiness). It comes out as quantitative, measurement-oriented, and standards-based. But experientially, a researcher sees the world as episodic, changing across time, and describes it interpretively and qualitatively. We all see it both ways. Sometimes our descriptions emphasize criteria and sometimes personal experience. We

BOX 3.1. Here

We are always somewhere. Wherever we are, we are always not just at but in some particular "here" that is not "there." We stand somewhere, sit somewhere. In words and abstractions (thinking, saying), our minds may wander from this gentle but unforgiving reality, but we cannot escape being in some here-ness, wherever we are.

We breathe the air here. This place enters us. We breathe in or do not breathe in the pollen that causes some of us hay fever in the spring. (And yes, we are always here at some particular time.)

Moment by moment, always, restlessly, we jolt, bump, jostle or caress the here-ness of here. We shed a tiny fragment of dead skin here, leave a footprint, snap this twig, swallow water from this stream, touch moss.

Living and dying, we participate in the great cycles of being. Ashes to ashes, dust to dust, some here receives us back into itself. And here nurtures or erodes us, even as we nurture or erode here's here-ness.

We breathe and eat here. What we eat, from here or there, was nurtured or torn from its locatedness somewhere—its being-there, its being in the here-ness of there. Ego-centric, we may think it made and made over for us, but it is made for us no more than we are made and made over, not just for ourselves, but for Being.

There is no exemption from being here, wherever we are.

Nor has here, in its here-ness, any exemption from our being here. It does not express feelings about our being here in words, in saying in any human language. Here expresses its relationship to us in continued capacities to be or be transformed, mute of language but not of being. It would be best if we could reconcile ourselves to the consequences of this brute fact—sooner rather than later. We leave a footprint in the soil here. We savor and swallow here the fruits of the earth brought to us from some here, some other sacred place. We inhale and exhale here, and clutter or clean the air that blows about the globe, taking traces of our here-ness everywhere.

The soil of here travels slowly. Water rises or runs through here's catchments to enter oceans or evaporate into air here. Here's air circles the earth, connecting our breath and fates to the breath and fates of every living thing and every other thing forever. Our doing—what is done—is done. We may want to but we cannot deny that we are here, that we were there, that we left a footprint.

(cont.)

BOX 3.1. *(cont.)*

And it is not just me here, but you and me, and you, and you, and you. . . . Like every living thing, I am embodied through acts of others, built from their genes. I jostle among others, endlessly nurturing or bruising, even where I mean to do what is best. We live and love in bodies in which we are smaller or bigger than others, more or less capable and caring than others, kinder or more dangerous to everything and everyone.

We are not just thinking and saying. We are not just doing. We are always relating, always connected to the earth and others. We are always, wherever we are, part of earth's flows, and the earth and what is in it are made part of the flows of our restless being by our being here. Though we may resist, resent or rejoice in it, we are part of a common humanity. Our lives make and leave marks on a shared earth, shared fates.

Source: Kemmis (2007). Reprinted with permission from Stephen Kemmis.

need to know about the kind of tree and its maturity and about your personal climbing tree. Both are good. Both are necessary. Both descriptions can be improved.

Criterial thinking calls for being explicit about the variables, the measurements, the sampling, and the cutoff standards to be used to get evidence for assertions. Criterial thinking emphasizes formal statements and explication. Often, criterial evaluation focuses on only a few criteria of successful performance, criteria such as worker performance, text comprehensibility, parent participation—measured simply. Many criteria are outcome variables. Criterial description relies on indicators of performance. We sometimes say, "The proof of the pudding is in the eating." According to this way of thinking, it is the outcome that counts.

There are lots of different ways of doing criterial research, most of them with focus more quantitative than qualitative. For example, an assessment system may be based on a single test of worker proficiency to represent the quality of all aspects of the work force. Researchers do that knowing from previous studies and experience that there often is a positive correlation among different indicators of program performance. So, many think that, if you measure one criterion well, it will tell you how well workers would perform on other assessments, on other criteria. The ranking is more important than directly measuring. That is the way the criterial researcher often thinks: It's better to measure a little well than to measure a lot poorly.

Looking ahead, criterial researchers conceptualize outcome levels, levels of confidence, levels of decision making. How high will the performance have to be for a certain decision to be made? They do not usually set such levels, but they would like their analysis to be that refined. What they may do is to take the forthcoming performance and compare it with a previous performance to indicate how the thing is working. Or they may compare the performance of the studied group with the performance of a control group. At other times, they leave it to experts to decide, after the fact, what the meaning of the performance is—but many of them dislike such subjectivity. Most criterial evaluators are happier when they can be explicit in advance about the level of success, such as using a level of statistical significance. An objective standard is wanted for deciding how the thing works.

What criterial researchers are most proud of is their measurement. They like to get numbers down on paper to show the performances of participants and beneficiaries. They analyze the numbers, sometimes in complex statistical ways, to show how things are working. They might show, for example, that—after adjustments for differences in prior standing and amount of assistance provided—the changes just made caused production to rise significantly. Sometimes that will be seen as increasing understanding of how the thing works.

But it takes more than that to conclude with some certainty that other things work that way, or that policy should be changed for future operations. For generalization, we need to study variations of the changes in a variety of situations. Seeking generalizations is pretty much the way of ordinary social science and policy study.

I started my career doing criterial research. When I did instructional research in the early 1960s, I was a psychometrician and an educational psychologist, and I only did criterial research. But I failed to make that research answer enough of the practical questions, so over the next 40 years, I slowly changed to being more of an ethnographer and case researcher. And I recognized this as more experiential work and called it "responsive evaluation." But here in this book we are calling it "qualitative research," and we are seeking activity more than merit.

Qualitative research is experiential, using personal judgment as the main basis for assertions about how something works. Because personal judgment needs to be based partly on personal experience, experiential research places heavy reliance on examining the personal experience of people being studied—manager experience, prisoner experience, the experience of others, but also the experience of the researcher. When possible, experiential researchers work face-to-face with the activity, with the problems, with the expectations and ambiguities and contradictions—sometimes immersed in them.

Usually, understanding grows deep through experience. Experience is universal. When your mother and father had you as a baby, they made a great contribution to the grand totality of experience. Your life experience is being added to the history of humankind. The fact that other people around you have different experiences does not make your experience less important. All count. And the typical is seldom more informative than the unusual.

In experiential research, standards are important even though they usually remain unspoken. Usually the standards are set intuitively and often separately for different people: how hard to work, how long to wait. These standards are based on past and current experiences of the people involved.

Yes, experiential research is relativistic research. It is situated research. It is common in daily life, in corporate life, in government life, especially for the most important matters.

3.3. EMPHASIZING PERSONAL EXPERIENCE

The more criterial the research, the more the emphasis is pushed away from personal experience toward standardized measurement and toward generalizable knowledge. Experiential research works to reestablish an orientation to the experience of individual persons, however large the group.

Of course, the researchers can go too far in individualizing or localizing the study. Community values need to be taken into account. The values of the people collectively, as expressed in district, state, and international documents, may be important in helping to learn how things work. Experiential research is not a commitment only to the values of the individual person but a commitment that the values of the individual person will be well considered.

In trying to understand how a corporate internship program worked, one researcher interviewed several interns. It was common for them to say things like:

> "I remember my interview for this internship. We had to prepare a personal statement and career goals. All I wrote was that I want to help whomever I am working for. I just want to help people to be better. That's what I am all about."

The speaker may have been sincere, but this is a promotional statement, promoting program or self or something else. It is not a statement about experience in the internship. Even if the interns describe in detail what they do, the data need a good deal of triangulation through observation, artifacts of accomplishment, and views of other people, plus skeptical interpretation. The best qualitative research, I think, is seldom about how people feel; it is about how things happen, how things are working. Happenings are experienced, and the researcher needs to probe the assertions until the experience is credible.

Experiential researchers seek multiple realities, the different meanings that different people give to how things work. They usually end up feeling that one reality is more pertinent or useful than others, but they try to display more than one reality to the readers of their reports, such as a nurse's reality and a patient's reality. Experiential research usually does not seek simplicity or the best explanation but a collection of interpretations.

How mainstreaming a child with disability was working in one primary school classroom in Ukraine was told by Svitlana Efimova and Natalia Sofiy (2004). (See more on the Ukraine study in Section 10.2.) They selected 8-year-old Liubchyk as their case, a boy with autism enrolled in a regular first-grade classroom. After observing him in his classroom, they went far and wide to make observations and interviews, connecting with other mainstreaming activities in the country. They interviewed people in teacher training and at the Ministry of Education. Box 3.2 records Svitlana's personal experience in Liubchyk's classroom.

Mainstreaming children with disabilities is a problematic situation, potentially an extra burden for the teacher. But this report showed that

BOX 3.2. Liubchyk's Classroom

I was visiting the first-grade room of the "Children of the Sun." Together, the children had chosen this title. They liked to say that they were the "Children of the Sun." On the classroom door were this title and individual photos of all the children.

It is 10:50 A.M. on a day in March 2004. Liubchyk is just coming in with his mom. She helps him take off his coat. Liubchyk is a slender boy, a tall boy, with fair hair and grey eyes. He is 8, a child with special needs. He first started preschool here in Maliuk School back in 2000.

Liubchyk goes immediately to the Reading Center. He stays maybe 3 seconds, then comes to the teacher's table. Ms. Halyna, the teaching assistant, comes across and greets him, "Good morning, Liubchyk!"

He cheerfully replies, "Halyna, at seven!" (which seems to mean that Ms. Halyna should remember to return home from work at 7:00). He takes several photos from the teacher's table and starts looking through them. Pointing to a picture, Halyna asks: "Who's that?" "Adij," Liubchyk answers. He starts saying the names of all the persons in the pictures. Then he puts the pictures back in the envelope and returns them to their place on the table. "Halyna, lunch too-welve," he says, pointing to the clock. "Yes, lunch is at twelve," Halyna answers.

The classroom teacher, Ms. Oksana, is working on mathematics with the group as a whole. The children saw Liubchyk come in, but were not distracted from their tasks. After Oksana gives the children small individual tasks, she approaches Liubchyk to greet him, "Good morning, Liubchyk." "Oksana, at seven!" he replies. "Please say, 'Good morning.'" He does. "Liubchyk, will you work here with us?" He says, "No," and goes to the Reading Center and starts turning the pages of the mathematics textbook. The group lesson goes on.

Source: Efimova and Sofiy (2004). Copyright 2004 by the Open Society Institute. Reprinted with permission.

the three teachers were managing the situation well, that the children were learning extra "caring skills" because Liubchyk was their classmate. They were learning how "this thing worked." The case study of Liubchyk helped readers understand how Ms. Oksana changed from being opposed to having Liubchyk in her classroom to becoming an advocate for inclusion.

And a few general comments: The purpose of qualitative research is usually not to reach general social science understandings but understandings about a particular situation. By understanding better the complexity of the situation, we should contribute to setting policy and professional practice.

We should look both for the general and the particular—as David Hamilton did (in Chapter 2) with the case of the chairs—but each of those aims wants to eat up all the budget. Good instruments are very expensive to develop. Good observations and interviews take lots of time. The things we want most to do leave little time for the rest.

Some people will say that collecting "experiences" is not real research and cannot help science. As Bent Flyvbjerg (2001) said, "They are wrong."

How is making professional insight more complex much different from building science? Experiential research can help a practitioner reconsider—during action—what needs to be paid attention to. New experience changes intuition. Formal knowledge can do the same, sometimes better. Professionals need both reason and intuition, criterial thinking and experiential thinking.

One of the epistemological strengths of experiential research is the belief that how activities work (activities such as campaigning and therapy) is situational. What the campaigner or therapist is doing is influenced by culture, the home environments of the people they work with, the conditions of the meeting place, and the personalities involved. Describing these describes how things work.

Experiential researchers sometimes use case studies to probe the meanings of situations and to report to readers the complexity of personal performance. Some of us try to extend to readers a vicarious experience of the activities, thus a better opportunity to decide in their own way how things work.

In experiential research there is a need for participants and outsiders to interpret what is going on. So the researchers present vignettes, pictures, dialogues for discussion, verification, and interpretation—seeking alternative meanings. What first appears as a subjective account of happenings—when triangulated and reasoned through by respected others—can become a trusted part of the report.

I have been talking about what all of you do every day, seeking to understand things, criterially and experientially. Doing formal research requires both, too. And each can be done with sensitivity and discipline.

3.4. MULTIPLE REALITIES

When you look at an apple up close, each eye sees something different. The left eye sees more of the apple's left side and the right eye sees more of the right side. You are not confused by the discrepancy. Your mind tells you that you are seeing the apple in three dimensions. Psychologists call this message from the brain "binocular resolution." It gives you the perception of depth.

When you and your friend go to a concert, you do not each hear the same thing. She says the music makes her think of her childhood, and you say the saxophone was garish. We do not expect people to hear the same thing; in fact, we feel enriched by the different perceptions, the different experiences people have, in the same place at the same time. We sometimes call it "multiple realities," and we feel a deeper hearing than we would with just one of us listening.

In qualitative research, many of us take a constructivist view that there is no true meaning of an event; there is only the event as experienced or interpreted by people. People will interpret the event differently, and often multiple interpretations provide a depth of understanding that the most authoritative or popular interpretation does not. There are multiple interpretations also, of course, of groups, motivations, accomplishments, and many of the phenomena we study. Readers sometimes can see more depth in our reports when we portray more than a single reality. Consider Box 3.3.

Akira Kurosawa's film *Rashomon* (1951) visualized an ambush of two travelers and four highly different versions told by the man and his wife, as well as by the bandit and a witness—a classic example of multiple realities.

3.5. BRINGING IN THE EXPERIENCE OF OTHERS

The new researcher sometimes makes the mistake of thinking that, although he or she is building upon the findings of other researchers, all the new thinking has to be his or her own. Actually, much good qualitative research greatly involves the thinking of others as data and interpretation. Thus the researcher is a listener, an interviewer, and a finder of the observations others are making. Long after formally reviewing the literature, he or she is finding relevant understandings from other research-

BOX 3.3. Moishe and the Pope

About a century or two ago, the Pope decided that all the Jewish people had to leave Rome. Naturally, there was a big uproar from the Jewish community.

So, the Pope made a deal. He would have a religious debate with a member of the Jewish community. If the representative won, the Jews could stay. If the Pope won, the Jews would leave. The Jews realized that they had no choice. They looked around for a champion who could defend their faith, but no one wanted to volunteer. It was too risky. So, in desperation, they finally picked an old man named Moishe, who spent his life sweeping up after people, to represent them. Being old and poor, he had less to lose, so he agreed. He asked only for one condition to the debate. Not being used to saying very much as he cleaned up around the settlement, he asked that neither side be allowed to talk. The Pope agreed.

The day of the great debate came. Moishe and the Pope sat opposite each other for a full minute before the Pope raised his hand and showed three fingers. Moishe looked back at him and raised his index finger. The Pope waved his hand in a circle around his head. Moishe pointed to the ground where he sat. The Pope pulled out a communion wafer and a glass of wine. Moishe pulled out an apple. The Pope stood up and announced, "I give up. This man is too good. The Jews may stay."

An hour later, the cardinals were all around the Pope asking him what happened. The Pope said, "First, I held up three fingers to represent the Trinity. He responded by holding up one finger to remind me that there was still one God common to both our religions. Then, I waved my hand around me to show him that God above was all around us. He responded by pointing to the ground, showing that God was also right here with us, in our midst. I offered the wine and the wafer to show that God absolves us from our sins. He pulled out an apple to remind me of original sin. He had an answer for everything. What could I do?"

Meanwhile, the Jewish community had crowded around Moishe, amazed that this old, somewhat feeble man had done what all their scholars had insisted was impossible! "What happened?" they asked. "Well," said Moishe, "first he said to me that the Jews had three days to get out of the city. I told him that not one of us was leaving. Then, he told me that this whole city must be cleared of Jews! I let him know that we were staying right here." "And then?" asked a woman. "I really don't know," said Moishe. "He took out his lunch, so I took out mine."

Source: Joke circulating on the Internet.

ers, practitioners, and members of the public. Qualitative research relies partly on the experience of others.

One of the best dissertations I have known was done by Tom Seals (1985; see Box 3.4). Tom was a doctoral student in counseling education and his research question dealt with therapists' conceptions of gender issues in marital therapy. As I saw it, his main method was to collect and compare the interpretations of fellow counselors, chosen because of their experience and expertise in marital therapy.

One way of looking at Seals's research was to say that he arranged a common experience (viewing his videotape of a marital counseling session) for a group of experienced professionals, then worked individually with them to get their interpretations. Some of them knew what a few colleagues were saying, but Seals was the only one who studied all of them, and he made his interpretations of the collection. It was a study heavily weighted by psychological theory, yet highly practical in its approach. He successfully brought together the immediate experience and the professional experience of others to complete his dissertation research.

Seals's study was an example of getting a huge amount of interpretive assistance. When you do a study that needs data from a great distance, you need to get help from acquaintances, family, and persons you employ. You need to think deeply about how to prepare them. It is not enough just to give them a copy of this book to read. You probably need to give them detailed instruction and to anticipate what could go wrong. It often is more work to train them what to look at and listen for than it would be to gather the data yourself.

Another kind of assistance of great value is to find a person already a part of the site at which you will be studying to brief you on how people there think things work, the ways things are done there, and who will be good sources of information and interpretation. Sociologists sometimes call these people "informants" (not meaning spies). As part of your report indicating methods used, you should speak openly about the help being given and gotten.

Qualitative description of how things work relies heavily on personal experience. The researcher usually has face-to-face encounters with the activity. Interviews are arranged to learn more about the experience of the participants. Episodic and situated description of the activity gives the reader a vicarious experience of happenings. The evidence for the researcher's assertions about how the thing works often includes much

BOX 3.4. A Study of Marital Counseling

Seals studied the conceptions of gender issues in marital therapy as illuminated in an actual case, that of Pete and Lisa, who had come to two of his colleagues for help with marital problems. He used one of their videotaped sessions with them as an exhibit to begin his dissertation research.

Interested in four theoretical orientations (psychoanalytic, family systems, behavioral, and existential-experiential), Seals hoped to make a theoretical contribution to counseling theory. Following his reading of Glaser and Strauss (1967) and impressed with their constant comparative method, he chose to follow a deliberately incremental approach to design and data gathering, particularly in introducing existing theory progressively through the study. Some people call that approach "progressive focusing" (Parlett and Hamilton, 1977).

He invited the participation of 16 marital therapists, selected so as to have four of each theoretical orientation. He had each therapist watch the tape as if they might be called in to help the counselor, then to prepare an assessment of problems and suggestions for assistance. He eventually interviewed each therapist, giving little focus to gender issues. The transcripts ran to 600 pages.

To work incrementally, he worked first only with the eight behavioral and existential-experiential therapists, interpreting their responses. Seals also employed a colleague to evaluate his ongoing interpretation of transcripts, looking particularly for omissions, additions, and distortions. Her comments were included in the data set as it moved through subsequent stages. Seals produced two synopses of the psychoanalytic and existential-experiential data, one an interpretive story of lifelong emergence of gender issues, tracing Pete and Lisa from the present on back to courtship and families of origin. The other was a taxonomy of therapeutic allusions emerging from the observations.

The eight therapists provided a comprehensive overview of gender issues in marital counseling, concluding that Pete and Lisa were experiencing predictable conflicts between men and women with normal gender roles in intimate relationships.

Seals was ready for further complication. He went on to the third group of four, the psychoanalytic, repeating the procedure but changing questions to address possible gaps in previous interpretations. Subsequently, the marital conflict appeared more to be something of a search for protection, searched separately by Pete and Lisa, after having faced inadequate gender identification in family-of-origin problems. The fourth sample did not add anything new. Although his two grand interpretations were at odds, Seals included both views in his conclusions.

Source: Based on Seals (1985).

description of personal experience. The evidence should be affirmed by repetition and challenge, much of it experiential. Qualitative research is a disciplined working through to experiential understanding, small amounts aggregating to larger insights.

This chapter has connected the reality of qualitative research with the reality of personal experience. The topic of the research is not always human activity, but the perspective is the human perspective. As soon as the writing starts to talk of variables, descriptors, scales, indicators, and attributes, then it is moving away from the experiential and toward quantitative thinking. Nevertheless, many qualitative designs include some quantitative thinking, bringing to it a certain depth. A different kind of depth comes from recognizing the multiple realities people have experienced. Qualitative researchers look for ways of gathering the experiences of others and finding still others to add new interpretations.

CHAPTER 4

Stating the Problem
Questioning How This Thing Works

Your research question should be more important to you than your research method. What you are studying should be more important than how you are studying it. Of course, some of us, maybe all of us, enjoy particular ways of seeking understanding of how things work. But our understandings would be fragmented and context-bound if we organized our thoughts around our methods.

As I write this book, I am trying to think of you and your situation. In certain ways, you are an expert. You have done some projects, maybe dozens. You are becoming more specialized in your field or taking on a new field. Some of you are thinking about capstone research for a career. Others are thinking about the steps of thesis research, maybe a dissertation. Some of the following chapters will deal with constructing a proposal and laying out a plan for data gathering and analysis, for thesis or capstone. These activities are going to make sense and go easier as you select the topic you will study. Bear in mind what poet John Moffitt wrote:

To Look at Any Thing

To look at any thing,
If you would know that thing,

You must look at it long:
To look at this green and say
'I have seen spring in these
Woods,' will not do—you must
Be the thing you see:
You must be the dark snakes of
Stems and ferny plumes of leaves,
You must enter in
To the small silences between
The leaves,
You must take your time
And touch the very peace
They issue from. (1961, p.)
> *Source*: Moffitt (1961). Copyright 1961 by Houghton Mifflin
> Harcourt Publishing Company. Reprinted with permission.

Many writers about qualitative research methods encourage new researchers to look at what is ordinary, look at it closely until "the ordinary looks strange." That means, choose a research question about something people know a lot about, then find connections and interpretations that help readers realize they didn't understand the complexities. If and when people criticize your study, you may find protection in the way that you have steered the research question into a new light.

4.1. FIRST THE QUESTION, THEN THE METHODS

What if we were to store in this corner all the things that we have learned by listening to our elders and, over there, all the things we have learned by surfing the Web—thus studying by two different methods. If you organize your research by methods (listening versus surfing), it will be a hodgepodge. Better, first, to ask what do you need to know; then, how to go about finding it. Better to organize by content.

Consider this. If your new cell phone shows a puzzling icon, you may ask your partner to explain it, or you may read the instructions[1]— two methods. Both are good research methods, but neither is likely to

---

[1] On Garrison Keillor's *Prairie Home Companion* show (March 9, 2008), it was said that to keep any personal messages secret, store them in a new folder named "operating instructions."

help you understand how cell phones work. Accumulating and storing information by subject matter, that is, by the content of the research question, is necessary for research—and for your use of it as well. You knew that. And now you know you may be spinning your wheels if you just love qualitative methods but have no idea what questions you might study using them.

Sometimes particular information is all that you need just now regarding your cell phone—not about cell phones in general. Sometimes it is just the opposite. When you decide which question to ask, then you decide what methods of inquiry to use. Whether intuition or reason tells you, you should think about what you want to know before you think about how to find out. Did I make that point already? Given that, I can think of two opposing points of view. We can set up something of a dialectic, an argument.

My office mate Iván Jorrín-Abellán (2008) said:

> It is quite difficult to be expert in several methods. How can we decide the best method without knowing some of them in depth? Sometimes our expertise in a particular method makes us select the method before the question.

The choice should not be limited to one's own expertise. You ask people with experience. You read. And you become more knowledgeable while the research goes along.

But Iván is right. All researchers are in training; even Galileo was. In their career they may need experience using both experimental methods and case methods. So they may design the next study partly for the purpose of getting better at a method. Your preparation for a career should include experience with various modes of inquiry. And a few of you could have main careers as methodologists, perhaps one of you specializing in one particular method, such as concept mapping (see Section 6.2). And maybe you will write chapters in handbooks about that method. It's not such a bad life.

Getting answers to substantive questions is not the only reason we do research. We do research partly to learn better how to do research. *Buscar ayuda buscar.* Seeking makes better seeking. So we will sometimes choose a method we want more experience with and will modify the research question to fit the method. Method before problem, sometimes.

The third point of view is that of Studs Terkel (1975) and Terry Denny (1978). They have said that many of the important stories are out there to be found—not always fitted to the etic issues you have in mind, but perhaps even more important. So they would encourage you to approach the scene with an open mind, and watch and listen, without much of a research question. It seems to me a good approach if you are rich or retired or a true populist like Terkel or Denny, but not so good for furthering a professional career. Later in this book we again consider giving a prominent role to the stories from the field—the patches—in shaping the organization of a final report.

For most of us, most of the time, the research problem should have first priority—but a question cannot be conceptualized without some thought of method and place of study. One cannot think deeply about the content of research without thinking of its meanings as studied one way or another. And the reality of studying it one place rather than others quickly forms in our minds (see Figure 4.1). In other words, first conceptualization of the study happens pretty much all together, the focus shifting from question to method to place and back to question, each time hopefully refining the idea. And the refining will continue well into the time you are gathering data and writing up patches for the report.

Most careers in research are defined by content questions, content such as care for people with Alzheimer's, computer-supported collaborative learning, or theater set building. The questions you raise will be stepping stones to your career.

To get and keep that career moving along, you shouldn't rely on research questions that are too broad, such as "How do children learn to read?" although that might help identify the child development or language arts territory in which you want to work. Your center pivot should not turn on trivial questions, such as "Did the boys or the girls read faster?" You should ask questions of substance:

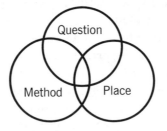

FIGURE 4.1. Simultaneous attention to question, method, and place.

- Are the concepts of "mainstreaming" and "pluralism" fundamentally opposed?
- Is it futile to try to integrate (beyond just mixing) "mathematical thinking" into the "pedagogical thinking" of teachers of mathematics?
- What are the personal and community values of the elderly women's chanting sutra groups of the rural South China coast?

And you should ask questions that have novelty, something of your own curiosities, eventually to link to what others have done, but something you can call your own. Some questions should be contentious (Wildavsky, 1995, p. 9). For your lifetime's work, your stepping stones should be carefully chosen.

For any one study, you may have just one main question, Research Question 1. You will be interested in other questions, too, some more abstract and some more particular, but one or a few questions need to be on target substantively (the right subject matter) and at the right level of specificity to guide the inquiry. In Figure 4.2, I have listed many questions at several levels, from general down to more situated. The ones toward the top are suited to a research career. The ones in the middle are about right for a dissertation, and the ones below are better suited to smaller studies such as course projects and preliminary studies. The questions toward the top are major but reach for too much intellectual territory for any one study. And at the bottom are the information questions, some of which will be important as part of a study, but not hefty enough to be the big Question #1.

All of these types of questions in Figure 4.2 have a place in a research study. But perhaps most important is the research question (one or a very few) used to structure the organization of the study. These few key questions are used to plan and carry out the study and possibly to organize the final report. The aim is to make some relationship or situation or phenomenon or trade-off more fully understood. These questions are not unlike basic research questions—but they are more focused, with special attention to contexts.

Developing the research question for a dissertation may require many pages of description, but description alone will not suffice. The questions may be articulated and interpreted using the aims and concerns of stakeholders of a program. From data gathered on each question, the researcher develops assertions or generalizations, possibly worded similarly to the original questions, but declarative rather than interrogatory.

Examples of TOPICS OR AREAS OF INTEREST (very broad)	• Upgrading the preparation of professionals • The social cost of meritocracy • The ethics of medical research • Advocacy for peace • The care and feeding of newborn infants
Examples of BASIC RESEARCH QUESTIONS (broad)	• What is the public support for making parks and playgrounds more child-oriented? • Why is drug rehabilitation not more effective? • Are the concepts of "mainstreaming" and "pluralism" fundamentally opposed? • How are major policy decisions made in collegiate athletics departments?
Examples of Research Questions for ORGANIZING A DISSERTATION	• How do teachers assess student art making in exemplary sites? • Does the heavy emphasis on marketing to youth in shopping malls bring in more shoppers? • Do organizational conditions facilitate or even allow a department head to be a moral leader? • How are war veterans contributing to the protection of rights of native Americans?
Examples of Research Questions for ORGANIZING A SMALL STUDY	• Is the fact that breeding standards are now set nationally affecting competition at dog shows? • Are attitudes toward obesity changing among young adults in this community? • Is increased emphasis on student test scores in this school an obstacle to teachers helping students improve self-concepts? • For professional staff members of these hospitals, what is the relationship between home residence and absenteeism?
INFORMATION QUESTIONS, too narrow usually to be a research question, but may be useful	• How effective at budgeting is the director? • Do drivers here understand how traffic volume affects global warming? • Of the total amount of class time here in these classes, what proportion is actually instruction time? • Given these rating scales, is there correlation between nursing quality and nurses' empathy toward patients? • In what ways have caseloads changed in the last 2 years?
IMMEDIATE PROBLEMS AND CHOICES, perhaps important, but not usually considered a research question	• What computer graphics software should be purchased? • How will the manager's work get done if that position is eliminated? • Should third-grade aptitude testing be ended here? • Is conflict of interest an issue regarding the appointment of the director's cousin to head community relations? • Does this textbook cover too many different things?

FIGURE 4.2. Six levels of research questions.

The research question helps you keep focus throughout a study. Still, it sometimes happens that you need to refine or even replace your research question during the study. That may be costly, but from what you learned in the previous pages, in qualitative research you may be wise to change the question. Even though brief, the research question tells better than the title of the report what you are going to do and, at the end, what you did. A research question or two or three may be among the important choices you will make in your academic lifetime.

4.2. LAYING OUT YOUR STUDY

You are going to be doing some formal research, maybe a lot of it. You have done some in the past, for term papers or department reports, looking up distributions, satisfying an assignment; but now the standards for organization, for connection with the research literature, are rising. I sometimes call qualitative research "disciplined common sense." You still will rely a lot on intuition, but you need to think ahead, to lay out a plan, even as you protect your spontaneity. Most of us need to get better organized, to find a better focus to our studies, to appreciate the situation in which we will be studying, to know something of what others have researched on the same topic. Organization of your study should start with a research question, but sometimes it starts with an episode, or what Luisa Rosu (2009) calls a "workable," a happening needing really deep thinking, needing microanalysis.

You probably know about how much time you will have to do the study, but it is hard to know how to design it so as to make the study big enough to earn the approval or credit you need and small enough to keep you from promising too much. A lot of the knowledge about design comes with experience. For now, you may have some idea of how many pages other people use to make such a research report, but that fails to tell you enough about how big and how small the coverage of your research questions should be.

You may have an idea of an instrument or procedure you would like to use, such as an attitude scale or someone else's oral history study, but that doesn't tell you how to write the research question or how much time to allocate to different activities. There is a lot of ambiguity at the outset, and it goes away slowly, but more quickly as you talk about it and try things out. A lot of trial and error. Sometimes you have to study what someone else assigns you to study, but even then, a lot depends on what you want to do.

Some studies are planned in great detail at the outset, and some are open and developing as the study goes along. Most faculty members and bureau directors think that, for your own good, you should make a strong plan. Along the way, some of them will encourage you to stick to your plan and—as you find out more of what can be learned—other advisors will encourage you to move on to another question or other complications and contexts. Think big, plan big, but do a small, well-contained study. Usually.

Sun Yat-Sen (1986) said, "In the construction of a country, it is not the practical workers but the idealists and planners that are difficult to find."

To get a suitable amount of data—aggregative data and interpretive data—planning can be difficult. Two years from now it will seem easier. You have to consider expectations of bosses and faculty members and others as to how much digging you should do and how much intellectual territory you should explore. But the size of the event or the territory is not a very good guide. You might do a study on what several international consultants have been doing in recent years and still end up with too small a study. Perhaps you just didn't find enough to make a good report. Or you might do a study on what one local consultant did during one week, and your study could turn out to be too big. Perhaps you reported so much detail that only two people will read the whole thing. So you need to get some idea as to how much readers will want to know and how much patience they will have in reading your stuff. Luckily, you have lots of experience as a reader. And you can get some advice from people more experienced, and you can try out your table of contents and some draft sections on a few thoughtful readers. It's something like coaxing an African violet.

4.3. A LIBRARIAN THINKING OF A DESIGN

Let us take the case of an inexperienced researcher, call her Marie, wanting to improve her skills as a workshop director. She decides it might help her to study a forthcoming computer-enhanced workshop for school librarians. She thinks about the workshop as a case to be studied.

Marie knows that school librarians routinely help children use computers for individualized projects on different topics. Her study could be an evaluative study, looking to see whether the workshop is of high quality. Or it could be a study of the homogeneity of teachers needed to make the workshop operate well. (For example, are there problems combining primary and secondary school participants, library assistants, and experienced librarians in the same sessions?)

Initially Marie wanted to find out those things about her own part of the workshop, thus to do an action research study (Chapter 9). But then she decided she wanted to study the workshop as a whole.

Let us say that Marie, a librarian herself, first identifies three research questions. Read them carefully. (I should tell you how to read?)

Are there conflicting beliefs among the participating librarians about project-based learning?

Are there competing rationales for helping students with web-based projects?

What coaching skills do these participating librarians bring to the workshop?

Reading them carefully, we see that Marie's questions are about the participants but not about the workshop itself. If she were to gather data on just these questions, it could be good but not a clear step to make the workshop the thing studied. And it might be too small a study to satisfy a curious reader. Those are three good questions, but unless Marie finds out more to report about the workshop, it probably will not be a good study.

You might say she should just change her focus from workshop to participants. But let's say that Marie wants especially to understand the pedagogy and curriculum of the workshop. For her, the workshop is the thing. She wants to know how this thing works in its situation.

So what are the ordinary things for Marie to find out? Most readers will be curious about the agenda, about the personal experiences, about the sponsors of the workshop, the financial considerations, social opportunities, and of course about the faculty. Most would like to know about the context or situation in which the workshop occurs. These seem to be good topics to consider in the study. But if each of the topics were dug into, she probably would have too big a study, a study too time-consuming to accomplish and too voluminous to read. (Don't we promote ourselves as curious inquirers and our readers as bright but busy people? Not always realistic, of course.) So Marie decides that her main research question should be:

What happens at the computer-enhanced workshop oriented to advancing the coaching knowledge and skills of the participants?

And as subordinate questions she plans to find out:

Do the participants form something of a "community of practice" to help each other learn during the workshop and possibly later?
What is the rationale of the planners of the workshop?

These workshop happenings and the rationale could make a nice little study, not big enough for a thesis or an internal evaluation study, just a nice little study. The questions fit together substantively. The happenings should be observed, but if she interviews those present, she can round it out and triangulate (Chapter 7). Some of the rationale can be learned from documents, but documents often do not tell enough, so she probably will have to dig into the rationale by asking the planners. For all these questions, Marie will be gathering mostly interpretive data but might have a small checklist questionnaire for participants, thus adding some aggregative data. This looks like what I like to call an "embraceable" study, something Marie can get her arms around.

In studying the workshop, Marie will also learn some things about the faculty, about how the workshop was advertised and financed, about the spaces and computers used, about the use of individualized training and suggestions for these librarians assisting other librarians, about a lot of things. And she will say a little about these things in her report, but she should use at least a third of her report to deal with her main research question and perhaps another third to deal with the two subordinate research questions. Marie probably should omit some of the good things she will learn in order to have a strong thrust or concentration on the research questions. Yes, she will trim away some good stuff.

Suppose midway Marie is tempted to add three more research questions:

How are recent developments in computer technology taken into account?
How does this workshop compare with another workshop offered these librarians?
Does the faculty understand enough about contemporary school libraries?

Each of them is an excellent question, but even one of them could be stretching the study too far. Adding all three in some depth probably would be too large a topical coverage even for a dissertation. The embrace would be lost. It is usually all right to change a research question a little, but to pursue well these last questions might call for three additional studies. Or she might be able to give a few hours and a page or two to each question, a mere arousal for her readers.

With the research question well in mind, Marie will do the study her way. Another researcher would choose a different research question and do a different study. For the vitality of the international community of researchers, it is important to have researchers selecting their own things to study and studying them in their own way. Still, with the experience and personal preferences that researchers have, it could be a mistake for Marie not to seek out a few from that community for advice.

Each time Marie modifies a research question, she needs to decide afresh whether the answers or stories or relationships she wants are something that people somewhere already know. (If yes, she needs to collect and interpret them.) Or whether the answers are not known by people but will rise out of the observations and analysis of the data. For example, if she wants to study what it is like to become a workshop director, then she will probably get good knowledge by asking people who are experienced directors. But if she wants to relate how directors make choices under stress, she probably will become better informed by observing them in stress situations. Where lies the knowledge? If she observes the directors, it is up to her more than to them to make the interpretations for her report. Of course she may draw a director or others into helping with her interpreting.

This is a major strategic choice: expecting the interpretations to come from the "data source" people (e.g., interviewees, authors) or expecting the interpretations to rise up out of your aggregation of scores and observations. I sometimes call the two *interpretive data* and *aggregative data*. If you interview participants having experienced a poor program, getting lots of quotes that you interpret as pertinent to your research question, we call them interpretive data. If you interview participants using the same structured questions for all and tally and analyze the results to get a sense of what is typical and what is dissimilar, we call it getting aggregative data. In leaning more toward immediate interpretation or toward aggregation, either way you are taking a step toward refining your research question. As indicated in the previous chapters, interpretive data find more of a home in qualitative research than in quantitative, but both kinds of data will be found in all research. You often cannot answer questions about how things work without using both interpretive and aggregative data.

4.4. DESIGN FOR STUDYING HOW THIS CASE WORKS

To design a study, I find it useful to lay out and rearrange the information domains and the research steps on a whiteboard, easy to stretch out, easy to erase. For Marie, some of the domains were: coaching skills, homogeneity of trainees, computer enhancement, and project learning. Then I collect these terms into boxes, figuratively, as in Figure 4.3, and then literally into file boxes. I call them "April boxes" because April Munson told my class that, for her, these boxes changed her research outlook from overwhelming into something doable. With pencil lines, I divide a large sheet of paper into six or eight boxes or more. I put all the contents of an information domain or topic into one box. Notice that I do not indicate here how I will get the data. Research methods come a bit later. Expanding and developing the research question comes first. And

Workshop
  Administration
  Rationale
  Risks
	Workshop curriculum
	  Coaching skills
	    Computer supported
	    Collaborative learning

Workshop staff
  Coaching skills
  Knowledge of computers
	Activities
	  Online orientation
	  Demonstrations
	  Role play
	  Simulated project
	  Break time
	  Trainee initiatives

Other
  Contexts (history, etc.)
  Budget
  Software
  Research on professional development
	Workshop trainees
	  Eligibility
	  Homogeneity
	  Community of practice
	  Beliefs about teachers

FIGURE 4.3. April boxes for Marie's study of a computer-supported collaborative learning workshop.

get this—some of the boxes (through iteration; Chapter 11) are likely to become chapter headings and topical sections in the final report.

Next, I actually label a number of green file boxes—mine are 4" × 9" × 12"—and start collecting definitions, explanations, transcripts, diagrams, and other things. When they are dialogues or stories that I think I might actually include in the final report, I mark them in a special way (sometimes needing to put copies in more than one box because I don't yet know where I will use them). I call these special dialogues or stories "patches," and I later claim that putting the patches together is an alternative strategy for writing the final report.

Next, Marie needs to think about data gathering. What methods have I already used? Which methods will I use most? I like to make a graphic sketch emphasizing my research methods this time. I often use a spatial graphic, such as the one shown in Figure 4.4. The hexagon in the middle represents the study. It represents what the researcher is going to do. Here we have indicated four data-gathering activities: observation of activities, interview, document analysis, and the brief study of minicases. There could be others.

The circles around the outside represent the conceptual territory inside which the researcher will be working. The larger circles identify the research question (and research related to it), the contexts, and the main information needed. The smaller circles represent the phenomena important to the study and some larger issues. By sketching out this information, the researcher makes a graphic plan for carrying out the research.

Marie chose to do a case study of a professional development workshop. For her graphic plan, the case is such a dominant idea (Stake, 1995) that we will change the graphic to represent the case with a heavy-lined circle, as in Figure 4.5. We will put the study activity within that circle. So we do it not exactly like Figure 4.4. Of course, you adapt it, too. Inside the circle design are spaces to guide Marie's data gathering. Three sectors have been marked for observations in three places. There could be more or fewer, of course. Then one middle-sized circle indicates a minicase that might help the reader understand the workshop.[2]

---

[2] A *minicase* (sometimes called an embedded case) is a case within the case; here it might be a workshop participant who illustrates a special problem or opportunity. Perhaps 5% of the final report might go to the description and interpretation of this minicase.

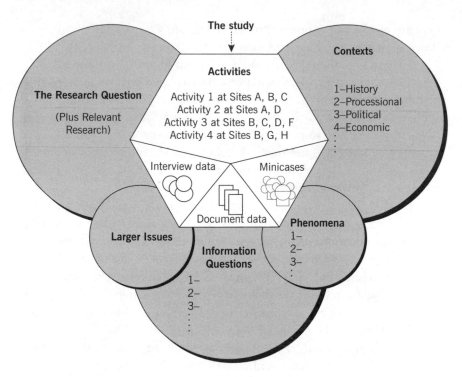

FIGURE 4.4. A graphic form for designing a qualitative study.

In Marie's study, there seemed time only for one minicase. The main artifacts and documents for Marie to review were—at least at first—the training materials and the statement of standards for school librarian proficiency.

For Marie's research, four contexts seemed worthy of examining: the history of this library, the national school library association, contemporary community support for school libraries, and research on professional development. And among all the information needed, Marie emphasized the backgrounds and the attitudes of the participants, the agenda for the workshop, and the hardware and software available.

As you know, one needs to have a research question and places to study it and some sense of how the needed information can be gathered. One will find stories, episodes, dialogues—the good ones I call "patches"—that will fit into one's boxes ready for interpreting the research question. (It may be necessary to get institutional approval for the protection of human subjects—Section 12.4—even before one knows

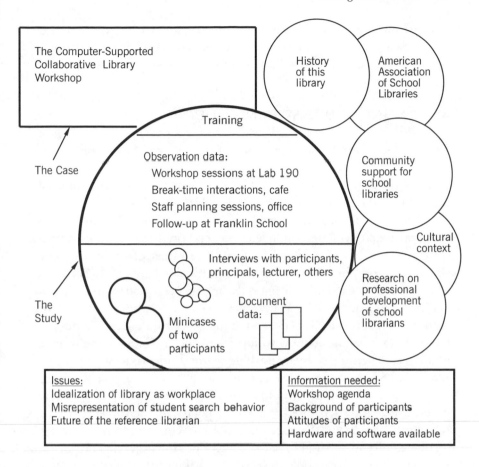

The Computer-Supported Collaborative Library Workshop

History of this library

American Association of School Libraries

Training

The Case

Observation data:
 Workshop sessions at Lab 190
 Break-time interactions, cafe
 Staff planning sessions, office
 Follow-up at Franklin School

Community support for school libraries

Cultural context

Interviews with participants, principals, lecturer, others

The Study

Document data:

Minicases of two participants

Research on professional development of school librarians

Issues:
Idealization of library as workplace
Misrepresentation of student search behavior
Future of the reference librarian

Information needed:
Workshop agenda
Background of participants
Attitudes of participants
Hardware and software available

FIGURE 4.5. Circle design of Marie's workshop study.

the situation well enough to create such a graphic plan.) The boxes-and-circle plan can be useful in conceptualizing the study during the remainder of the study, with modifications expected as the work progresses.

There is a risk that the plan will become a mechanism that interferes with the open and interpretive stance taken by the qualitative researcher. Marie's question is about how the workshop operates, both practically and conceptually. She needs to be thinking about what is happening here, using her intuitive curiosities, as well as gathering observations to analyze. And such curiosity needs to extend to what can be read on similar topics in professional and research documents and to thoughts of how the library and teaching professions can profit from knowing even a little thing such as how this workshop worked. Of course, if Marie does not care much about understanding it deeply, it can't be expected to be good research. These graphics may get in the way, but they also may stimulate your expansion and deepening of the research question.

4.5. RAISING AND ANSWERING QUESTIONS

Dissertation research and other kinds of research can be pursued with a variety of methods, in a variety of places, and with a variety of targets. Figure 4.6 indicates some of the different targets to study (without needing to know the content of the research question).

The 3 × 3 arrangement here is of no consequence. The list of nine was drawn up to counter a frequent expectation that qualitative studies are mostly studies of personal feelings. The target of the study sometimes will be a phenomenon, either a particular happening, such as a dedication of a particular memorial, or a general happening, such as dedications of memorials. Many phenomena are cultural, such as the tendency of dentists to be male, and many are natural, such as a possible tendency in Indiana for snow to fall following the blossoming of magnolia trees. There are so many possible methods for studying any area of research. Following are some examples.

As an example of a study of personal relationships, one could examine how generation-separated siblings get along with each other. For many relationship questions, the researcher looks for correspondence, how two attributes vary together (as one increases, does the other increase also?). For example, we might study how cooking habits and gender are related, such as was the stimulus for the 2003 Swedish motion picture *Kitchen*

Studying a case	Studying a phenomenon	Studying a relationship
Studying a policy	Making a comparison	Evaluating a program
Studying a distribution	Inferring a generalization	Doing a natural experiment

FIGURE 4.6. Some main kinds of qualitative research studies.

Stories. Many studies of correlational relationships (correspondence, covariation) are more quantitative than qualitative, but correspondence is important everywhere. As the moderator interrupts the debaters, do the claims become more strident? Or a correspondence between exercise routines and gender finding that, at one exercise spa, water aerobics was more popular among older women than older men. We could treat that same spa-specific, age-specific phenomenon as a gender difference or as a correspondence between gender and routine.

Policies, either informal habituations or formal requirements, can be studied: in terms of difficulties in changing policy, as manifestations of political values, as having costs and benefits, and in many other ways. In policy study, quantitative studies outnumber the qualitative. Comparisons are attractive because they are so simple; for example, "Which are the better telephone marketers, men or women?" Comparison questions are central (not surprisingly) in comparative research, such as the Tobin–Wu–Davidson (1991) study of preschool children in Japan, China, and Hawaii. Comparisons are often macroanalyses, with focus on population criteria, outside the box of most qualitative researchers.

Evaluation studies are different only in the sense that the research question raises the question of merit or quality. We usually think of distribution studies, inference studies, and experiments as quantitative, but distributions can be nonquantitative patterns, such as distribution of attention by a nurse. And inference studies can be any studies in which we carefully monitor influences and contexts so that a generalization can be drawn. Natural experiments happen when an event occurs, such as an extended power failure, and the changes in activities are carefully recorded. Each of the nine target studies of Figure 4.6 can include both qualitative and quantitative work, making them "mixed-methods" studies in which more than one method is used to examine the very same content (see Section 7.4).

No matter which methods are used, research is about trying to make sense of important questions. The main question, the research question, seldom can be asked well in one sentence. When you propose research—for a contract, dissertation, or any other—you should take several paragraphs or several pages to explain your research question. Mine (Stake, 1961) started with "Do learning curves on small tasks provide parameters that add more about scholastic aptitude than we get from conventional standardized tests?" You can guess that I needed several pages to explain what that meant. How about yours?

CHAPTER 5

Methods
Gathering Data

Qualitative researchers seek data that represent personal experience in particular situations. Many qualitative data look like these three:

1. A campus official said, "This is a pretty new camp, but we're good."

2. In cadence, over 200 young voices shouted out:
   I will be—a good sport—at all times!
   I will conduct myself—with decency and honesty!
   I will do my best—to get along with others!
   I will have pride—in myself!
   I will put forth—my best effort—in all competition—and always compete fairly!
   I will walk tall—talk tall—stand tall!

3. Staff members did not receive paychecks until Wednesday of the third and final week. And there were payroll paperwork errors. Although they were informed of the pay schedule when hired, on Thursday the staff members were tense.

Many qualitative data are personal happenings in time in a place. These three would be included in further analysis if they were pertinent to the research, if they helped move toward understanding how something works or does not work. Here the thing being evaluated qualitatively was the National Youth Sports Program. How did it work? Did it work differently from camp to camp at the 170 participating colleges?

Of course, qualitative researchers use all kinds of data: numerical measurements, photographs, indirect observation,[1] texting, for example; whatever clarifies the picture of what is going on. They review documents[2] and gather artifacts (Hodder, 1994). Clearly, many qualitative data do not fit easily into statistical analysis, although the researcher could classify each datum according to a categorical scheme such as "youth initiated, coach initiated, and college official initiated." We talk about analysis and interpretation of data in Chapter 8. Our attention here is on finding and recording data.

A few "raw descriptions" may appear in the final report; most will be winnowed, sorted, and further interpreted. The choice as to which patches are worth keeping and, later, worth inserting into the report is not easy. At the time it is encountered, the qualitative researcher makes some guess as to whether or not a particular one is valuable enough to hang onto. Later he or she will make further decisions as to its value. Does it help us understand and talk about the research question? Some of the sorting is arbitrary, but experience makes it less so. You cannot keep every datum, and some data that later would become valuable will be passed by. Still, the newcomer to research has been making choices like these in ordinary living for years, and gradually he or she will refine the habits of recognizing good stuff for qualitative inquiry.

As indicated early in Chapter 4, methods for gathering data are selected to fit the research question and to fit the style of inquiry the

---

[1] Once, indirect measures were popularly known as "unobtrusive measures." It soon was realized that unobtrusive observation can be an invasion of privacy (see Section 12.5); also Webb, Campbell, Schwartz, and Sechrest, 1966, and Stephen Baker's 2008 book, *The Numerati*, on personal data collected for marketing.

[2] Lindsay Prior (2004) ended his handbook chapter on using documents in qualitative research with these words:

> In all of my research settings documentation was central. Yet while I was in those settings I often regarded talk and interaction as somehow more real and more deserving of attention than the paperwork that was lying around and about me. Nevertheless, if I were nowadays asked to give just one piece of advice to the novice researcher, it would be as follows: look at the documentation, not merely for its content but more at how it is produced, how it functions in episodes of daily interaction, and how, exactly, it circulates. (p. 388)

researcher prefers.[3] Some qualitative researchers give high priority to open-ended questions, minimizing categorical and yes–no questions, and these have value when it is the interviewee's story or the program history that is needed. But many questions and views needed to develop a research question have to be composed by the researcher to get information. Such questions are illustrated in Box 5.2 (p. 96). Any one of the questions could be followed by a yes–no probe, such as "Have you opposed that development?" or a more open-ended question, such as "Tell me how that got started." Qualitative research will find a place for any method sooner or later.

Many well-developed methods for qualitative research already exist. Many are catalogued in handbooks, textbooks, and journals such as *Qualitative Inquiry* and on the Web (Denzin and Lincoln, 2006; Johnson and Christensen, 2008; Seale, Gobo, Gubrium, and Silverman, 2004). Using a method, protocol, or approach that has been tried and found useful repeatedly can save time and increase meaningfulness. But few will be just what the researcher and the research question want. A review of the literature should give some attention to how other researchers gathered data for similar research questions. The emphasis in this chapter is on the strategies of data gathering more than on particular techniques.

5.1. OBSERVING

Many qualitative researchers prefer observation data—information that can be seen directly by the researcher or heard or felt[4]—to other kinds. The eye sees a lot (and misses a lot), simultaneously noting who, what, when, where, and why (as newspaper people are supposed to do) and particularly relating them to the story or the assertions forthcoming—that is, to the research question. The story, assertion, the boxes, and

---

[3] Many formal proposals for research include a methods section. It should describe what will be done rather than teach what certain methods do. The methods section or chapter of a final report should provide detail as to what was done (and therefore cannot be completed before the research is completed).

[4] The apprentice qualitative researcher asks, "How do I do it? What do I look for?" There are no simple answers, no dependable generic checklists—for good reason. Observation methods need to be made particular to the situation. One of the most thorough writings on these techniques for qualitative researchers is by Patricia Adler and Peter Adler (1994).

even the research question will change as the study goes along, and the mind's eye changes, too. Sometimes the observation goes like Box 5.1.

The research question here was about the quality of the National Youth Sports Program (NYSP). The observation in Box 5.1 is about the role of discipline in the program, a theme running through the study. Here and generally, I find something of a dialectic, a tug of war for attention, between the observations and the theme. And both influence each other. New data sometimes have an effect on the research question, often making it more complex. And as the theme matures, the meaning and value of individual data change. When I first heard the youth chanting (see the beginning of the chapter), I thought of it as telling that they acknowledged the importance of being "good sports," and later, with many more data, I saw the chanting more as militarization. Interpretation is a part of observation and continues to reshape the study along the way. In Chapter 7 we look at how triangulation is used to strengthen the meanings we give to things and to tease out new meanings.

In the field, some observation data are immediately seen as valuable. At an Indianapolis federal office, I asked an official if she thought of herself as a bureaucrat. She said, "I'm not a bureaucrat." "What are you?" "I'm a Hoosier." I knew almost immediately I would repeat that patch in my report. As I said earlier, I call those data that immediately, by themselves, seem relevant "interpretive data." And those that become relevant only when mixed in with lots of other data are "aggregative data." The repetitious ways in which Mr. Hussein talked about physical and mental conditioning are qualitative aggregated data. A researcher designs the observation procedures differently when expecting aggregative more than interpretive data, or vice versa. Can you say how? Do you relate it to microinterpretation and macrointerpretation?

Four of us on the NYSP evaluation team each visited a participating college campus. Perhaps we should have, but we did not use an observation form to observe NYSP activities.[5] We relied on the researcher as the instrument, capitalizing on intuitive ability to see in depth, to recognize the influence of context, to probe, and to progressively focus. A fixed instrument is sometimes constraining, although usually better at maintaining focus and facilitating aggregation of data. We thought that

---

[5] One example of such a guide is shown in Figure 8.1. Even when major sites are identified in the design and formal observation guides are used, the researcher usually needs to be gathering data informally in the spaces around the sites, among people not anticipated as data sources, in the media, on the Internet. Serendipitous data will identify gaps, add information, and enrich the interpretations.

BOX 5.1. Martial Arts

At 10:00 A.M., into the gym. Then it takes 15 minutes more for the boys to get into places. They seem unable to form ranks, to have anything of the perspective that good things can happen if they follow the organizational plan of the teacher. Makir Hussein takes them individually and places them in a spot in a matrix five by five. Mario occupies the back row, right corner spot, Mark creates a spot behind the group, Peter lingers at the door.

This is the wrestling room, about 30 × 40, high ceiling, warm. Sponge pads cover the floor. Its cement walls and severe box shape and use designation give it a stark look, maybe even a combative feeling.

The formation is fluid, swirling, kids melting to the floor pads, pursuing minor variations of fake fighting. (After the morning pledge, the kids had vigorously responded in cadence form, as led, "I WILL NOT" "FAKE FIGHT" "I WILL NOT" "FAKE FIGHT".) At any one time, maybe half have drifted off spot. With half the group in place, Hussein brought them to attention to try to keep them in ranks but that quickly wears off. Hussein offers a maxim: "If you can keep quiet, you can do anything." A couple of boys exceed the allowable dissension. They are sentenced to the hall, soon to be hauled off to the office by Mark.

Now with all approximately organized, Hussein brings them to attention again, and quickly into the side spraddle hop. Everyone responds in vigor, shouting out the count for every second move. The spirit of excess remains.

Now, in the fourth of ten sessions, a small amount of background to authenticate the martial arts. The boys seem not to need it, but they listen up. I am unable to comprehend quite a bit of what Hussein has to say. He delivers it something as would my stereotype of a revivalist preacher: "For this is the Way [pause] Life is Lived. The Body's the Line between [pause] the Heart and the Way. [pause] DO YOU COPY?" I have trouble believing that the youngsters are copying what I cannot— but they sound out in unison, as I am moved to myself, "Yes!"

Focusing it is, but not spellbinding. A voice instantaneously asks, "Mr. Hussein, can we get a drink?" This is a tough choice for Hussein because he wants total concentration on the task at hand, has finally got to Square One, but, with room temperature not far from 100, faces the possibility that he will turn down a request for water just prior to a twelve-year-old passing out. This time he holds out, but he will not at the next plea, 20 minutes from now. A bit more philosophy in his mixture of army dialect, revival, and street language: "Knowledge . . .

(cont.)

BOX 5.1. *(cont.)*

love . . . grounded support . . . balance . . . personality . . . power . . . knowledge." Then, "AM I RIGHT?" "RIGHT!" "ARE YOU READY TO MOVE ON?" "YES!"

He takes them through five or six moves. Left fist forward. Right foot back. Left knee bent. One move at a time, repeated twenty times, describing it at a shout, then counting off the repetitions. His movements are elegant, disciplined, visually arresting. The boys keep an eye on him, feel their bodies making some such move, then carry it out extravagantly, outside the rim of demonstrated action. Few of them lose sight of interesting challenges to right or left.

"Okay, this is the alphabet. Each of these moves is a letter. What do you get if you put them all together? You get words. These are the moves that make up all the martial arts: Korean, Japanese, Chinese. Basically, they are all the same." He puts Sylvester into a position, fist forward, elbows out, leg back. "Balance . . . ready . . . hard to move him . . . heavy like a mountain." Again and again, the group follows Hussein, moving forward and back, intent, wanting it as an individual, not yet showing much group adherence.

"Mr. Hussein, can we have a drink?" Although several of the boys answer, "No," Makir Hussein cannot refuse again. First he urges: "Forget about time. Make your own conditions. Forget about water breaks." But he allows their disbanding and the last ten minutes of the class is lost.

letting each observer write up the story of his or her visit independently would help the reader see the uniqueness and similarities of each camp. Still, observation forms might have helped us focus on the NYSP issues, issues such as:

1. Which ethic is picked up by the youth, the "striving" or the "winning" ethic?
2. Is the heavy involvement of police as coaches an asset or an obstacle?
3. Does the national office (National Collegiate Athletic Association; NCAA) stress compliance or independence in the operation of the camps?

Designing even a small data-gathering instrument is a big job, often not done well. Will its scores represent what they are supposed to represent? Will the survey in Box 5.4 (p. 100) really represent competitiveness? Many researchers today are so caught up in getting "human subjects protection" approval that they spend too little time getting the data redundant and targeted on the research question. Each revision of a main data-gathering approach should be reviewed by other researchers and piloted, not using the people who will provide the final data to be analyzed, but people like them. The numbers in the pilot trials do not need to be large, but care should be taken to ensure that respondents understand what is being asked and that the data will fit into the analyses planned.

An active form of observation is *participant observation* where the researcher joins in the activity as a participant, not just to get close to the others but to try to get something of the experience they have down on paper. The pioneer anthropologist Bronislaw Malinowski (1922/1984) was keen on this approach, encouraging us "to put aside camera, notebook and pencil, and join in himself in what is going on. . . . Though the degree of success varies, the attempt is possible for everyone" (p. 21). But Clifford Geertz (1988) and others have been critical that we are too quick to presume that our participant experience approximates theirs. And to presume that we have not altered their experience by being there. You recognize why it is difficult for an adult to be a participant observer in a youth camp. An adult might profitably do participant observations there—but extra caution is warranted. Sharon Merriam (2009, p. 126) and Uwe Flick (2002, p. 141) offer an evolving view of this method.

One of the largest worries of a new researcher is making an accurate record of what is happening. I sometimes think he or she worries too much about the accuracy. Yes, it has to be right, but there is more than one chance to get it right. The first responsibility of the observer is to know what is happening, to see it, to hear it, to try to make sense of it. That is more important than getting the perfect note or quote. Much of what we put down is an approximation that we can improve upon later—if we have a good idea what happened.

The new researcher looks for safety in audio or video recordings, failing to appreciate how much he or she has to know in order to edit the transcript, failing to know how flawed the mechanical record often will be. Some researchers can use recordings effectively, but many cannot. What you have to do with observation—with and without recording—is to work at it, practicing, modifying, to see what you can do well. You have to expect to practice your data gathering repeatedly before actually gathering data. Get a coach. Tape yourself. Do the same with interviewing to train yourself to be a minimally proficient data gatherer. It gets better with experience. Still, some very good observation data are turned in by first-time researchers.

5.2. INTERVIEWING

Interviews are used for a number of purposes. For a qualitative researcher, perhaps the main purposes are:

1. Obtaining unique information or interpretation held by the person interviewed
2. Collecting a numerical aggregation of information from many persons
3. Finding out about "a thing" that the researchers were unable to observe themselves

The first and the third are tailored to the individual person and often should be conversational, with the interviewer asking probing questions to clarify and refine the information and interpretation.

If there is expectation that one or several interviewees will produce quotable materials, then the interview should be tailored to what is special about that person. Although the interview usually will be structured by the issues of the researcher (etic issues), it sometimes is better to ask an open question ("What was your experience early on?"), letting the interviewees just comment or tell stories (structuring them around their own emic issues).

If the responses to the questions are to be tallied (for example, finding 17 playing, 9 not playing), then the questions should be uncomplicated and put to all the respondents in the same way. (Such effort at repetition is usually called semistructured interviewing.) It sometimes is difficult connecting simple questions to a complex research question. Many complicated questions do not lend themselves to numerical aggregation. As part of the evaluation of NYSP, we asked local directors such open-ended questions as shown in Box 5.2.[6] Even though we planned

---

[6]Thoughtful opposition to open-ended questions has been expressed by David Silverman (2000, p. 294).

BOX 5.2. Interview Questions for an NYSP Camp Director

1. Are the major decisions of this program made in terms of what is best for the youth?
2. Are the aspirations of NYSP unrealistic, or perhaps too modest?
3. Is there a good balance in the camp between sports participation and nonsports instruction?
4. Do your coaches feel that your camp is too much like school?
5. Have steps been taken to ensure that your coaches follow good exercise routines?
6. We have learned that some camp staffs do not have the skills to help acquaint youth with career and educational opportunities. Is that a problem here?
7. Some community and campus leaders have spoken to us about the importance of NYSP experience in establishing the reality of being on campus and raising aspirations regarding higher education. Is that happening to the youth here?
8. Do you try to provide instruction using a participatory mode, with "hands-on" tasks leading to experiential learning? Are kids used as leaders?
9. Are your instructors and coaches required to submit lesson plans at the outset of summer activities? What might cause a plan to be rejected?
10. Many of the camps work to have the youth move about at breaks between activity periods quietly and in formation. Many make the disciplining of rule breakers well known to other youth so that others can learn the consequences. These are examples of a structured disciplinary approach, a "tough love" approach, helping the youth understand and live within a rule-based society. Is this your disciplinary approach here?
11. What has caused you to expel youth from participation? Tell me an instance.
12. What is your policy regarding admission of youth with special language needs and those with social, mental, and emotional problems?

our questions in advance, we did not ask them in a structured way but more as a topical conversation with probing. Note how these questions emphasize the operation of the program more than the effects on the youth. We did not compose the questions until we knew quite a bit about camp operations.

These questions are similar in form. Usually we mix the item types to relieve the boredom a little—getting the redundancy we want often gets boring. We did announce in advance something like: Since we are visiting so few camps, we need to be redundant in order to have confidence in our findings.

These were interpretation questions. With most groups I find eight to be about the right number of interpretive questions for an hour. We did not ask for stories directly, but we got a few, useful for our NYSP report. In other studies we need to ask for information about personal background, tenure, size of university, neighborhood—but we had that already.

It takes a really good interview or survey question for most interviewees to get deeply into the complexity of the thing being studied. Sometimes it helps to have exhibit questions, which we will talk about next.

5.3. EXHIBIT QUESTIONS

Especially with interviews, but in surveys as well, we can sometimes push respondents to sharper concentration by asking them to examine and respond to a specific statement, a story, an artifact, a quotation, or some such. Questions 6 and 10 in Box 5.2 are exhibit questions. We give respondents something to examine and draw out a recollection, an interpretation, perhaps a judgment. Several questions may follow the exhibit.

In a qualitative study of professional development in Chicago, our exhibit was a teacher retention situation described by a school principal. It is shown in Box 5.3. Several of the urban-school interviewees reading it remarked that the situation could not happen in their systems but that they did in fact have some ways of encouraging a weak teacher to move on. The most important data were the praise they gave teachers for caring personally for students and the confidence they had in being able to help teachers teach better.

BOX 5.3. Exhibit Question

Here is a scenario written by a principal having to reduce the teaching staff by one. Please comment on how it relates to your own work situation.

"We're in a budget crunch again. I have to let a teacher go. It's never easy. I'm having to decide between two teachers to let go. They both have issues. One is an older teacher. She has been here for years. She has always been a tough disciplinarian, and it's caused problems with parents in the past. But tough discipline isn't always a bad thing. The problem is she has a bad temper. She has been known to scream and yell at the students. She has thrown chalk and erasers. She has also been very resistant over the years to any kind of curricular change. She uses didactic, "drill and kill" methods—and she assigns lots of homework. Her student test scores are always fairly high, and every year or so you have a parent coming in saying that she has absolutely worked miracles with their child. But the majority of her students are terrorized.—The other teacher is incredibly well-liked by almost all her students, but she's just not a very effective teacher. Her students love her and they love all the fun projects she does. But somehow the popular projects don't translate well into achievement scores. The other teachers are critical of her because her classroom is loud. Her students cause problems walking to and from class. The other teachers have to step in and reprimand them. And her students are more likely to cause discipline problems on the playground. I have been in a real bind over which way to go. We struggle to maintain annual yearly progress, so I'm leaning towards keeping the one more effective instructionally, but in the long term, I'm not sure that's a good investment. If I worked with the younger teacher on her discipline and paired her with a more effective teacher, she might improve. On the other hand, she might not have what it takes to be a good teacher."

With this exhibit question, our respondents helped us understand how dissimilar to this their own staffing situations were and also how much they valued teachers who cared about the children as children. We learned about their confidence in building up the skills of teachers who were ineffective in instruction. The exhibit question stimulated some good answers from our Chicago respondents.

5.4. SURVEY

A social research survey is a set of questions or statements or scales—on paper, on the telephone, or on the screen—usually asked the same way of all respondents. The data are turned into totals, medians, percents, comparisons, and correlations, all fitting nicely into a quantitative approach. But qualitative researchers often save a part of their inquiry for quantitative survey and aggregated data. The advantages are that surveys can draw from a large number of respondents.[7] We used a 72-item survey—a small part of which is shown in Box 5.4—to learn how the NYSP youth, ages 10–15, perceived the 5-week experience. The response categories we offered formed a Likert scale, running from "strongly agree" through "neutral" to "strongly disagree."[8] The 13 aggregation statements here have a single focus, derived from the first issue about the program's competitive ethic, so a single score might be given for the section, a "competitiveness" score. In many qualitative studies, the survey items are interpretive items, each to be considered separately, such as:

1. Bickering, cheating, and making folks feel bad are pretty common at NYSP.   SD D N A SA
2. Coming to NYSP makes it pretty hard on my family.   SD D N A SA
3. During the last 30 days, on how many days did you have at least one cigarette?   0 1–2 3–9 10 or more

5.5. KEEPING RECORDS

Maybe you are already doing it. If so, good for you. All researchers, young and old, should keep at least one journal, better two or more (Silverman, 2000, p. 191). One of them can be a cell phone or iPod.

---

[7]In a procedure called "item sampling," with several hundred respondents, the total pool of questions can be divided up into subsets for a third or fourth of the total respondent group.

[8]I dislike the Likert scale, preferring more pertinent response categories, such as running, for example, from "none" to "many" or from "never" to "all the time," but respondents are acquainted with the Likert categories. Often, whether the respondent actually agrees or disagrees is not as high-priority information as whether or not the condition is high or low.

BOX 5.4. Part of the NYSP Youth Survey

B1. The coaches give most of their attention to the "stars."   SD   D   N   A   SA

B2. The coaches praise children when they play better than other children.   SD   D   N   A   SA

B3. The coaches make sure children improve on skills they are not good at.   SD   D   N   A   SA

B4. The coaches yell at children for messing up.   SD   D   N   A   SA

B5. Trying hard is rewarded.   SD   D   N   A   SA

B6. The coaches encourage children to help each other learn.   SD   D   N   A   SA

B7. The coaches make it clear who they think are the best children.   SD   D   N   A   SA

B8. The coaches encourage students to try their best.   SD   D   N   A   SA

B9. Children are encouraged to work on their weaknesses.   SD   D   N   A   SA

B10. The children really work together as a team.   SD   D   N   A   SA

B11. The children help each other to improve.   SD   D   N   A   SA

B12. Coaches pay most attention to the best performers.   SD   D   N   A   SA

B13. Doing better than other children is important.   SD   D   N   A   SA

SD, strongly disagree; D, disagree; N, neutral; A, agree; SA, strongly agree.

That one may be for your daily living, to keep track of phone numbers, addresses, Internet information, reminders. Then get another journal each time you start a research project, easy to write in. (If you want to be nice to yourself, get a Moleskine.) Here you should make notes about everything in the research: contact information, calendar, bibliographic references, risks; get it all in one place. In the same journal, put your ongoing speculations, puzzlements, and ponderings. For example, "Was she formerly a hospice worker?" Or "Shouldn't the job of research be to make recommendations?" Or "If you quote the interviewee *exactly*, doesn't it often make him or her look bad?" Write down your concern. You will need some of them later. The observation in Box 5.5—a patch, a "keeper"—was written up later from my journal, when we were evaluating NYSP, something probably to include in a report.

In the following months, we continued our field observations and survey work, analyzing the results, interpreting the issues, and preparing a report. Toward the end of the contract year, we heard from the national director that our evaluation would not be funded for the second and third years. We sent a couple hundred copies of our Year I report to NCAA headquarters but got no reply. Their office was moving from Kansas City to Indianapolis.

In this chapter I have identified four types of data-gathering methods. There are many methods within these types and other types. This book was not intended to be a menu of research methods. (That kind of help can be found in such books as Johnson and Christensen, 2008, and Bickman and Rog, 1998.) As conceptualized in Chapter 2, the most valuable instrument for qualitative research is the researcher—experiencing an event or listening to a person with special experience or browsing through records. This personal research needs to be planned and structured, yet open and adaptive. Most of the time, the research question is the compass point more than a standardized procedure. To be sure, strategy and technique are important.

BOX 5.5. Field Notes, NYSP

It's an elegant hotel in Kansas City. The three of us from CIRCE introduced ourselves individually to the several members of the Advisory Board we didn't know—a cordial moment—before taking chairs against the wall. It was our first opportunity to observe an Advisory Board meeting.

We had the agenda on our laps and were surprised when the National Director opened the meeting with a request to Chuck, the senior *internal* evaluation person, to describe the progress of our *external* evaluation project, now 5 months old. We were unaware that our work would be discussed and unprepared to participate.

Chuck said, "The researchers from CIRCE visited 20 of our 170 campuses last summer, surveying the students, interviewing the coaches, counselors, administration and campus officials. They had some serious data-gathering problems." This latter was news to the three of us. Since Chuck was the liaison between the Advisory Board and the CIRCE team and had participated in access arrangements and some summer feedback, we had talked with him frequently but had not learned that someone had seen flaws in our work.

The National Director and Chuck and the three of us were Caucasian. The Board and the 10- to 15-year-olds at the sports camps were predominantly African American. One Board member, James, asked Chuck, "Were the problems a matter of insensitivity to Black children and their parents?" Chuck said, "That seemed to be part of it."

James turned to us and asked, "Did you ask our children racist questions? Did you invade their privacy?" I tried to think what he could be talking about. In a whisper, I asked Kathryn and Rita if they knew. "No." "No." So I said, "Most of our questions were drawn from surveys of children used before in research projects. They were piloted at trial sites." I could have said that we had sent them in advance to project headquarters for review.

James said, "But you asked what their mothers thought, not their fathers. Why not? You asked children when they had last smoked a cigarette." "That's true. Part of your program is drug and alcohol education. We needed to know something about the frequency of smoking of the youth because, according to the National Center for Alcohol and Substance Abuse, the proper training depends on frequency of use."

Carswell said, "I wasn't aware that this was information *we* wanted. Don't you find out what it is your employers want to know?" He went

(cont.)

BOX 5.5. *(cont.)*

on to elaborate as to how things worked in the business world and drew supportive comments from other Board members.

I said, "As you know, we have a contract to evaluate this program. This first year we are concentrating on the children. Next year, on the staffs on campus. And in Year Three, on the national organization. The contract was based on our proposal, which outlined the data we would gather but did not detail the instruments and observations we would use. You Board members reviewed and approved that contract."

"You may have signed a contract," Carswell said, "but you apparently don't realize you work for us. Now if you are expecting to continue this research next year, you'll be asking what *we* need to know." The admonition continued, partly on how contracts should be negotiated; then questioned our fieldwork again.

James said, "Apparently one of your people insulted our students, claiming that they couldn't read. What kind of training do you give your people?" "I'm sorry. I don't know what you are talking about. Chuck, do you know?" "Yes, it's true." The National Director said, "I'm afraid we've run out of time. We need to go to my office where the photographer is waiting to take the annual picture."

We sat stunned while they filed out. I asked Rita, "Could this have something to do with Chicago?" She said, "I think there was some problem there. Harriet [our assistant] arrived with the questionnaires for the Notre Dame kids, same questions, of course, but wrong names. The Chicago Director (who seemed surprised we had come that day) said something like, 'Oh, we can just have the kids write their own names at the top.' And Harriet said something like, 'No, we need to be completely sure the names are legible. Some kids don't write very clearly.' And the Chicago Director said to Harriet something like, 'So you think our kids can't read! It's insulting for you to come in here and confront us this way.'"

CHAPTER 6

Review of Literature
Zooming to See the Problem

The most common format for a proposal to do research, as well as for a report of research, calls for a review of research already done. A review is almost universally required for a dissertation. In some places, graduate advisors require a draft of a review of literature as part of the dissertation research proposal submitted before a preliminary oral examination. A passing mark at that examination usually constitutes approval of the research topic plus the committee's assurance that the candidate is ready to undertake the research. The review of literature is considered evidence that the doctoral student has sufficiently examined the theoretical writing and research publications as a conceptual base for the proposed study. Many advisors have considered this literature review more as a "qualifying examination" than as the beginning of a study of a particular research question. That is an important difference for reading this chapter. For you other readers, you seldom will have such pressures to comb the literature, but you too will find that efforts to organize a bibliographic context will help you understand the problems early and help you interpret the findings later. It may be worth the effort.

6.1. REFINING THE PROBLEM TO BE STUDIED

Which came first, the chicken or the egg? Which comes first, the problem or the literature? For describing the research, we talk about the research question first, but the question would not exist without at least a scattering of "literature," including ideas from the classroom, documentaries, personal experience—informal, as well as formal, literature. Often the patterns of ideas of various leaders, such as Albert Shanker, teachers' union founder, and Peter Drucker, social ecologist, give shape to the early collection. But before that, the interest in a literature would not exist without an intellectual curiosity, without at least a small realization that something was worth studying. Similarly, with actual development of a review of literature, the researcher goes back and forth, thinking about the problem, taking note of what others have done, acknowledging the refinement of the research question during the study, and seeing new ties with the literature. It's back and forth, iterative.

One or more broad fields of scholarship and professional expertise are seen as a platform to build upon. To review the literature, both the doctoral student and seasoned researcher are expected to recognize key precedents, listing appropriate citations and at least, for some citations, some mention of the content. Broad fields are broken up into subfields, mapped out (for the review, as in Figure 4.3, I draw boxes on a sheet of paper, subsequently making smaller boxes and moving to larger paper) and carefully identified, and the best-known writers are named, quoted, or cited.

A few years ago, for her dissertation research, Juny Montoya Vargas studied the law school curriculum at University of the Andes in Colombia, at which she was a faculty member. It could have been called action research. What she called it was "critical study," meaning that she took a point of view—in this case, democratic values—as a framework for evaluating what the law students were being taught there. In her opening chapter she drew from the literature to extend the view of her research question. Following tradition, for her second chapter, she reviewed the literature, dividing the writing pertinent to her study into these 16 main parts (boxes, topics):

Critical theorizing and researching
Quality of critical research
Validity of politically committed research
Ethical responsibility in values-committed research
    Professional legal education
    Purposes of law school
    Legal education as general education

The liberal university as an ideal
    The law school curriculum, core versus periphery
    Coverage of rules versus teaching lawyering
Legal education in the civil law tradition
Legal education in Colombia
Evaluation orientations
    Democratic evaluation theories
    A rationale for democratic evaluation at this site
    Evaluation as education for democracy

In all, she cited 111 studies but drew most from perhaps 20 authors, spelling out certain of their positions. For example, she wrote:

> Gutman (1999) argues that although the university is not the place for basic moral education, there is a kind of moral education that the university can and should undertake: students can learn "to understand the moral demands of democratic life" by "learning how to think carefully and critically about political problems, to articulate one's views and defend them before people with whom one disagrees." (Montoya, 2004, p. 29)

As the researcher, she laid out an intellectual playing field on which the research game was to be played. The dimensions of the playing field had not been defined for her, although she had had advice here and there. Some mentors do set boundaries. Part of the implicit challenge of graduate study and of study leaves is for the candidate to decide what constitutes an appropriate literature, sometimes stretching and collapsing boundaries.

6.2. CONCEPT MAPPING

A qualitative researcher needs to represent one or more main concepts, particularly for planning the study but also to assist interpretation along the way. Frequently a researcher fails to find relevant research literature in other disciplines because he or she has not sufficiently considered that other disciplines use different terms for the same concept. A concept map may be helpful in recognizing literature in alternative fields.[1]

---

[1] Not all advisors and directors support the search for corresponding literature from fields afar. The more that the research is emphasized as belonging to a specialization or to a community of practice, the less useful interdisciplinary literature may be seen as.

Sometimes a concept map becomes sufficiently refined to be inserted in the final report. Many maps are just informal sketches, sometimes a cliché, merely boxes connected with arrows and words to make a sentence. A map should be more than that. Representations that display the parts are analytic. In some instances, a concept such as "grief and grieving" will be the target of what is studied, and the writings of people may be gathered and plotted to give an idea of the conceptual spaces encountered. The map may be formalized, developed from standardized ratings ("Is grief more like anger or loneliness?"), perhaps using multidimensional scaling (Borg and Groenen, 2005) or structural conceptualization (Trochim, 1989). Such programmatic sampling and analysis are needed if the researcher intends to publish his or her concept of a subpopulation, such as funeral directors or media production staffs. Qualitative researchers are more likely to portray the conceptualization informally, such as for professional discussion, than formally, in the form of scientific knowledge.

As an informal guide to planning (Novak and Gowin, 1984), the concept map can be sketched out on a whiteboard, easily changed, identifying various ideas related to the concept. Technically, to call it a map, we expect a distance function, with close proximity indicating ideas closely associated. And we expect a territorial function, with area indicating importance, as shown, for example, in Figure 6.1, a concept map for the topic of this book, "qualitative research methods." The plotting of the map could be dimensional, such as plotting "particularization" versus "generalization" on the horizontal axis and "personal versus impersonal" on the vertical. But most conceptual structures can be mapped on two-dimensional paper or whiteboards only by minimizing dimensional meanings.

In Figure 6.1, the sizes of the ovals indicate importance, and the distances between ovals indicate the closeness of association. You might wonder how "causality" could be plotted on a map for qualitative research methods. It is at the furthest distance, small in importance, but it is there because some qualitative researchers will present causal inferences in their studies. But it is also there because the concept of causality needs to be talked about when talking about qualitative research methods. None of that is clear from the map, is it? This is not a rich information map, too crude, but perhaps a step toward finding ways other people would define the concept. The map says much less than the list presented in Box 1.2. In what way is the list better than the map? How does a map differ from a table of contents?

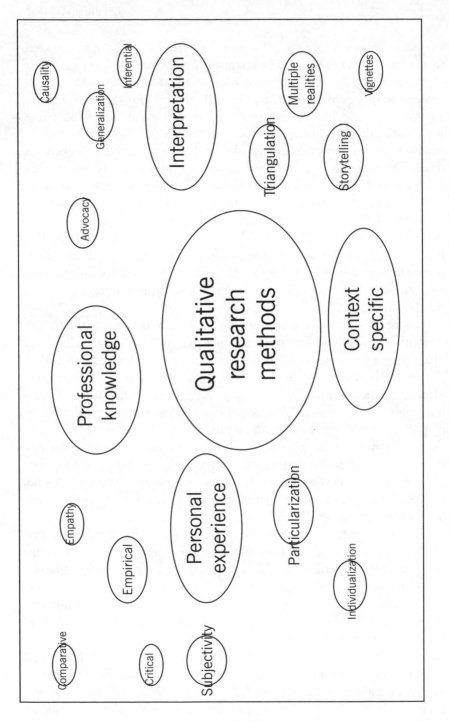

FIGURE 6.1. A map of the concept "qualitative research methods."

The concept map in Figure 6.2 shows a scattering of subconcepts or elements, all a part of the meaning of evaluation of teaching on campus. Here the distance and territorial functions were not considered important.

6.3. REPRESENTING THE FIELD

Some literature reviews are undertaken to represent the field—the field (or fields) containing the research question—a topical field such as "return of dropouts to formal education" or "geriatric care in refugee camps." Do you have such a field yourself?

An important distinction among literature reviews has been made between those called *systematic* and those called *conceptual* (Kennedy, 2007). Systematic is used to mean that an attempt has been made to find all the studies that examined a particular causal relationship. Yes, a causal relationship. An example would be seeking to know whether increased management attention to factory working conditions causes higher productivity.[2] There are different definitions of the two primary variables, management attention and productivity; the boundaries of the literature are far from fixed, but if the attempt has been made to be exhaustive, the review is said to be systematic. All others are classified as "conceptual."

Of course, in the usual meanings of these words, all "systematic" reviews are conceptual, and all conceptual reviews are systematic, to a certain extent. But sometimes we leap to make words say what we want them to say. The terms *systematic* and *conceptual* are arbitrary and should not be taken too seriously. But the two review styles do aspire to different ideals.

As pointed out in our first chapter, causal studies are not attractive to many qualitative researchers, seeming to them presumptuous and decontextualized. As curriculum researcher Mary Kennedy (2007) pointed out (during the George W. Bush presidency), the definition had political connection with the No Child Left Behind act and debatable claims that U. S. Office of Education policies were based on research.

---

[2]This is an actual literature that centers on recognition of the "Hawthorne effect," getting short-term gains from modifications of the assembly line (Franke and Kaul, 1978).

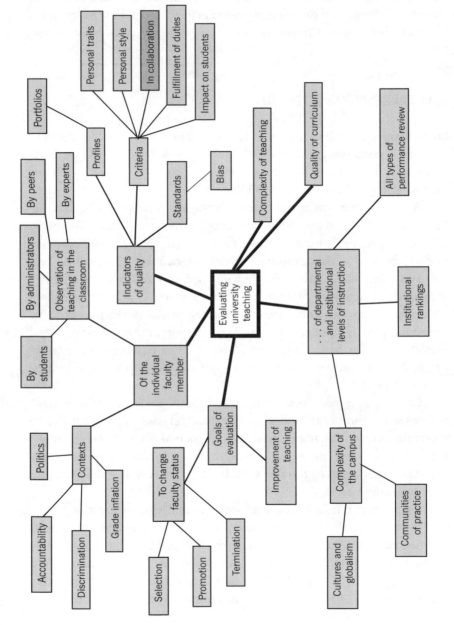

FIGURE 6.2. A map of the concept of "the evaluation of teaching on campus."

Kennedy criticized those who use the term *systematic* as treating statistical knowledge with higher respect than professional knowledge
(which she called "lore"). Setting aside this bias, we cannot but admire
those who work hard to build new research on the totality of previous
researcher accomplishments.

Some literature reviews aspire to maximize the broad and complex
conceptual standing of the research question. With a large number of
citations and working across four disciplines, Juny Montoya Vargas
aimed at this. Such a conceptual literature review is an attempt to bring
together writings on diverse matters related to the coming study's phenomena. It is a search for contextual relationships. It is the territory cov-
ered by a concept map. The conceptual review perhaps should be more
concerned about extending understanding into different fields (such as
politics, culture, and leadership) than in finding all past work examining
a single causal function.

Both conceptual and systematic reviews are challenging tasks,
answering different questions. The systematic may offer greater contribution to researchers in a developed field of research. The conceptual
may offer greater contribution to seeing the complexity of a professional problem. It seems important for those about to do dissertation
reviews of literature to choose between emphases on being complete and
on being broadly connected. Qualitative research is broadly connected
across the contexts of human activity. Speaking to researchers about the
2008 financial crisis (a context), Saville Kushner said:

> The significance of contemporary change for us and our role has just inten-
> sified. This is not to say that as we work to our contracts trying to under-
> stand and report on health projects, curbside safety projects, regional devel-
> opment initiatives and the like, that we are bound to report on the origins
> and impact of the contemporary crisis. But we should keep a weather eye
> on changing relationships between state and professions, shifting public
> attitudes and tolerances, emergent ways of thinking about social invest-
> ment and the moral obligations of government at all levels. This is the
> context to our work, and it is, at the least, prudent not to ignore it.

Kennedy (2007) encouraged researchers to set boundaries for a
search, especially for systematic reviews. Criteria for starting dates, language, and methods may be set. But it is often sufficient to indicate to
readers roughly what was searched and what personal criteria of relevance were used. Often the review will be enhanced by having another

researcher (or panel) review the search and selection criteria and think deeply, partly to comment on omissions. Criteria should not come first. The search should have begun long before the research question was worded and should continue until the report is circulated. Certain books, authors, and movements will be impetus for the study, but each may be augmented, sometimes replaced, as the study moves along. Qualitative research seldom is an engineering masterpiece; it is organic, and the tendrils of its reviews of literature shoot far, and sometimes wither.

6.4. BUILDING UPON THE NEARBY STUDIES

A slightly different choice to be made is between whether or not to allot most of the pages of the literature review to carefully unpacking the nearest writings (perhaps eight, or more, or less), the ones that most closely relate to the forthcoming research. This approach lends itself to the researcher's nourishing his or her still-forming ideas. And later, in the research report, it contributes more, in my view, to helping the reader understand the nearby conceptual space of the study.

Juny Montoya Vargas, having identified over 100 relevant research articles in 16 main topics, wondered how to distribute them across 60 pages of literature review. Of course, she did not know how many pages or articles there would be when she outlined the review, and she knew each topical "box" (Figures 4.3 and 8.2) would get some pages. But what would be the organization within the box? Consistency might have had her continue with conceptual subdefinitions of "critical theorizing" and "liberal university," two of her boxes. But she moved, as most of us would, to identifying the most insightful writers, a few or quite a few, within each box—for example, Joe Kinchloe and Peter McLaren in critical theorizing and Amy Gutmann in liberal higher education. Montoya Vargas gave them a little more prominence than others in the two boxes.

I encourage the researcher at least to consider going further, perhaps to give half the space within a box to paragraphs most illuminating the background for the present study. For Montoya Vargas it might have been to give three pages for the main 16 writings, or perhaps five pages for the main 8 writings. In other words, to write much more deeply about Gutman's view of the liberal university and to drop 50 or 80 of the citations. Clearly, that would be more "conceptual" than "systematic," but it might be a better stimulus to her later interpreting.

To illustrate this approach, let's take a passage from the book *Marking Time* by Paul Rabinow (2008). In this book-length essay, Rabinow—an anthropologist studying within the genomic biosciences community—claimed that his discipline (anthropology) was out of touch with contemporary epistemology and needed an overhaul. He developed his ideas by drawing deeply on the thinking of seven writers and artists whom he particularly admired, namely, John Dewey, Michel Foucault, Jürgen Habermas, Paul Klee, Niklas Luhmann, George Marcus, and Gerhard Richter. *Marking Time* is more than a review of literature, but Rabinow's style shows us one way to deal with literature. He was making his assertions through what had been said in his pantheon (see Box 6.1).

It might have been long coming to Paul Rabinow's mind that the ordinary rules of anthropology, as he had learned and practiced them, perceived the observer and the social system observed as relatively fixed. And gradually he knew that epistemologists were treating knowledge as ever under construction and increasingly challenged. Perhaps he had moments of epiphany, but even those would have flattened over time. And, perhaps gradually, he came to the assertion that part of the work of the anthropologist is to study simultaneously the observer (the anthropologist) and the field of anthropology.

What the researcher will write about his or her perceptual progress in conceiving the study will not be a map of actual progress. One's own reasoning is not transparent, even to oneself. And one needs to write to accommodate the backgrounds, values, and "adaptabilities" of the readers. One needs to invent a story, an itinerary, a construction of assertions that leads a reader to discover his or her understanding. For *Marking Time*, Rabinow chose to step through, to layer up, to string together, a few of the most pertinent views of his fellow philosophers.

In the excerpt in Box 6.1, from a chapter on observation, Rabinow posted the thoughts of George Marcus (and Pierre Poreieu) to make the point that, even as researchers live ordinary time-pressured lives, they still perceive their work and scientific truths more or less as fixed in time, outside of history, and capable of being nailed down. But Rabinow went on in subsequent sections, drawing particularly from social systems theorist Luhmann, to say that even mutations and kinship systems will be seen differently from place to place and time to time and that social science too needs to stop fighting evolution.

The fast-changing field of genomics is not yet a useful model for professional study and qualitative research. But the way that Paul

BOX 6.1. Pressures of Time

George Marcus (2003) astutely raises the issue of time, or better timing, in ethnographic research and writing, in an article entitled "On the Unbearable Slowness of Being an Anthropologist Now: Notes on a Contemporary Anxiety in the Making of Anthropology." Although Marcus is concerned with the profession of anthropology, and the production and dissemination of ethnographic texts, the topic of time pressures certainly arises in the biosciences as well. Marcus's article provides an excellent starting point for further questioning, further inquiry, and consequent reformulation of questions.

Marcus opens his article with a quote from an essay by Pierre Poreieu (1990) entitled "The Scholastic Point of View":

> In contradistinction to Plato's lawyer, or Cicourel's physician, we have all the time in the world, all our time, and this freedom from urgency, from necessity—which often takes the form of economic necessity, due to the convertibility of time into money—is made possible by an ensemble of social and economic conditions, by the existence of these supplies of free time that accumulated economic resources represent.

Few, if any, molecular biologists or active anthropologists would ever imagine today that they had all the time in the world to do their work, to produce results, and to have them published. In the life sciences, the ferocious, ceaseless, and ever more accelerated competition for priority makes this view of the leisurely pursuit of truth strictly unimaginable. Normatively, however, Bourdieu's claim that scientific truths are timeless has its own plausibility. Who discovered, published, and patented the sequence of the BRC1 gene matters only to the individual scientists (and their universities and companies). The discovery itself remains without historicity, at least for those who hold a realist view of scientific truth. A mutation is a mutation is a mutation. The traditional work of anthropologists fell, in a different manner, under that normativity of timelessness, as long as anthropology could maintain that the object of study (whether culture or society) was out of history or at least operating on a radically different temporality from that of the anthropologist in her modernity. A kinship system is a kinship system is a kinship system. Given this self-understanding, "anthropology could confidently insist on standards of research performance that valued deliberation, patience, and a stable scene and subject of study." Such a position has not disappeared, but is under renewed strain today.

Rabinow and others have used the literature to facilitate their study—empirical and philosophical—can be a model for qualitative researchers. The proximity of a few individual past researches to the present inquiry could be a better guide to page allocation in the review of research than it has been, extending the view of the problem. But it may be outside the rules at your place.

6.5. FINDING THE LITERATURE

For research writing, it is clear that much of the relevant literature will also be research writing, mainly that in refereed journals. It used to be that the journals were printed on paper and available after publication in bound volumes at the library. And that seemed where to look.

For one searching for literature on a particular topic, it becomes apparent that there are reviews already done on many topics and that there are journals of reviews. For the topic of "nurses' attitudes toward obesity," one can find the review by Ian Brown (2006). For research on "personal trust," one can find the review by Megan Tschannen-Moran and Wayne Hoy (2000). Such reviews are specialized in certain ways, and so often not fitting well what the researcher has in mind; but sometimes they are a gold mine.

A review of literature should draw not only from journals but also from other print and nonprint sources. Some of the search should be spent in dissertations, government and institutional reports, lecture series, and conference presentations, partly to gain a better understanding of communication that occurs in different venues.

It is possible to make reports of research appear more sophisticated than the research that occurred. And it is to be expected that the research that occurred was more complicated in some ways than the report portrays. Monitoring the quality of representation in reports is seldom considered of high importance in the research community. Some members acknowledge the slippage.

Beyond slippage: Lying, cheating, plagiarism, and endangerment of human subjects—upon investigation—should result in professional censure. There are misrepresentations in research reporting that are considered serious, such as failing to indicate personal relationships between researcher and supposedly independent interpreters. There are many omissions, hyperbolic descriptions, and careless editing of transcripts that are paid little heed. Not all researchers are saints.

The Internet[3] has become a great aid to research, particularly the search engines of Google. Some websites are interactive, providing opportunity for sharing research interests with other researchers.[4] But there are problems.[5] In most domains, monitoring of the quality of reports is lax. Should a researcher be censured for citing a poor-quality study? The ethic of most of the Internet is promotion and diversion, characterized by overlap and boundlessness of information sources. Gresham's law says that bad money drives out the good,[6] and the same may be true of information. Still, enormous banks of mostly good information are available now that were not available to researchers 20 years ago. Wikipedia is a valuable resource, in spite of the potential mischief of open editing. Wikipedia information begs to be checked, doubted, presented with caution. Triangulation is as important in learning from these sources as from our own face-to-face data sources.

---

[3] The much smaller, once-microfiched ERIC information system preceded the Internet. It was shunned by many researchers because it had low standards of admission and weak checks on credibility. But it contained, and may still contain, good information that still needs checking. Its federal support was diverted more for political reasons than because of its usefulness.

[4] At least for a while, look for Web 2.0 on Google; also Ebsco, Scopus, InfoTrac, and Google Scholar.

[5] A fine essay on Internet use for qualitative research was written by Annette Markham (2004).

[6] From Wikipedia (October 2, 2002) we learn that the concept of the bad driving out the good can be traced to ancient works, including Aristophanes' *The Frogs*, where the prevalence of bad politicians is attributed to forces similar to those favoring bad money over good. Aristophanes wrote (405 B.C.):

> The course our city runs is the same towards men and money.
> She has true and worthy sons.
> She has fine new gold and ancient silver,
> coins untouched with alloys, gold or silver,
> each well minted, tested each and ringing clear.
> Yet we never use them!
> Others pass from hand to hand,
> sorry brass just struck last week and branded with a wretched brand.
> So with men we know for upright, blameless lives and noble names.
> These we spurn for men of brass. . . .

CHAPTER 7

Evidence
Bolstering Judgment and Reconnoitering

We usually start our research having some idea of how the thing works. Whether it is software or a professional training program or the relationship between anesthesiologists and surgeons that we will study, we seldom go into it cold. We have some notions or expectations of what we may find out. Gradually, we become more and more confident that we will have something good to say about how the thing works. We will say it with confidence if we have good evidence. The evidence doesn't make it true. The evidence makes us confident that what we are thinking is right. We use evidence not only for bolstering our assertions but for updating our design and refining our data collection.

We could say that all our planning and data gathering is to obtain good quality evidence. That probably draws too much attention to the evidence and not enough to the interpretation of the evidence, but it implies what we already know, that evidence can be of poor quality and evidence can be of good quality, and good is better.

> Actual evidence have I none,
> But my aunt's charwoman's sister's son
> Heard a policeman, on his beat
> Say to a housemaid in Downing Street
> That he had a brother, who had a friend,
> Who knew when the war was going to end. (Reginald Arkell, in Bartlett
>   1968, p. 965)

Quality of evidence is a concern for reasoning in general, in all human affairs, including the attainment of understanding, making priorities, and choosing a course of action. As humans, we reflect upon experience, we gather and analyze information, we ponder and put meanings together; in other words, we synthesize. As researchers, we become persuaded which assertions will be the more dependable, and we counsel others to help them choose confidently a course of action. We are preparing evidence and understanding for users of research, the practitioners and administrators and policy makers. As users, to act with caution is important, and to wait for confidence is very important. We need to think through what evidence means in terms of user confidence.

In law, probative evidence is evidence that has the effect of proof. Teeth marks are evidence of a bite. According to *Black's Law Dictionary* (Black, Nolan, and Nolan-Haley, 1990, p. 555), "probative evidence is evidence that induces conviction of truth. It consists both of fact and reason co-operating as co-ordinate factors." If the evidence is probative, then finding it essentially eliminates doubt.

In a 1994 paper on the synthesis of evaluation, evaluation spokesman Michael Scriven attempted to guide program evaluators in that huge, final, procedural step of putting all the evidence together to describe and declare the merits and shortcomings of the evaluand. He urged design of evaluation studies to minimize bias by minimizing the role of human judgment. He would have us rely on probative reasoning. He explained that the evaluator should identify a small number of critical, objective criteria that would be seen and accepted generally, by the relevant users, as proof that the program was acceptable or not acceptable. Reasoning would be needed to select the criteria, but the evidence should be straightforward, he said, needing minimal judgmental interpretation.

The field of law takes that approach, defining the commission of a crime, or the exercise of a contract, or the execution of a deceased person's will, as resolved and legalized by meeting a small number of criteria. Lawyers and judges call these necessary and sufficient criteria, "elements." Take murder. First-degree murder. Generally speaking, the four elements are: (1) the killing of a person (2) by another person (3) who had the intent to kill (4) with premeditation. Just four elements must be present beyond reasonable doubt.

Evidence is defined in *Black* (1990, p. 555) as "any species of proof, or probative matter, legally presented at the trial of an issue, by the act of the parties and through the medium of witnesses, records, documents, exhibits, concrete objects, etc. for the purpose of inducing belief in the mind of the court or jury as to their contention." The interesting thing pointed out here is that the evidence itself does not resolve the issue but advances one belief over others in human minds. Evidence is presented to convince human juries and judges and guide their judgment. They then issue a verdict.

A court trial often has the appearance of an exercise of personal judgment. On television it appears as an emotional event—histrionics mixed with forensics. But dispassionate workings of the law have reduced many legal proceedings to a rubric, checking off a set of standardized elements. Another example: To establish the validity of a will, the attorney must show five elements: (1) the intent to transfer property, (2) the capacity to write the will (a sound mind), (3) the will in writing, (4) the decedent's signature, and (5) witnesses to the signing. The legal transfer of complex property has been reduced to a relatively simple technical matter, but the evidence still must be judged relevant.

Such formal protocol is essential to the vitality of the law. But is such reduction of social process otherwise in the best interests of society? Should a will be allowed to perpetuate a house of prostitution? Should a will be allowed to leave the state with expenses that the decedent should have provided, such as the care of his or her young children? Should a will be allowed to violate human rights principles? There is rationale and precedent for what the law allows, but one of the costs of reducing the law to elements is a restriction on the exercise of societal aspiration. Qualitative research could be, but should not be, I think, so technical, so objective, so uncaring.

In pharmaceutical research, in trials of new drugs, the publicized evidence of effect often comes from randomized group comparison with a placebo group. A fully tested drug is considered safe for uses controlled by doctors. Not everyone agrees that such evidence is sufficient, even when the testing follows scientific rules. Are pharmacology and the law good models for finding evidence of good professional practice (House, 2006; Sloane, 2008)? I think not. The criteria for social policy are much more complex. And, with exceptions, past controlled experiments of teaching, social work, and management have produced too little evidence (Walker, Hoggart, and Hamilton, 2008). History has not yet found workable social prescriptions based on sampling and independent of contexts. The evidence is unbearably light.

7.1. EVIDENCE-BASED DECISION MAKING

In academia, in professional practice, and in business and government today, there is widespread advocacy for evidence-based decision making (Cook, 2006; Denzin and Giardina, 2008; Lipsey and Cordray, 2000). That advocacy honors technological thinking and disdains intuitive thinking. One quickly understands that many of its advocates are speaking of evidence in the form of objective, science-driven, action-determining knowledge more than as material for user judgment.

Thinking this through, it will be useful to distinguish between facts and rationales. The common concept of evidence is as determination of fact. Did the student pass the course? Does the new photocopier jam paper more than the old one? Was community participation influential at the time? With reference to taking action, many questions are decided in binary fashion: yes or no. On time or late. Guilty or not guilty. In pharmacology, we think of sufficiently or insufficiently tested. Pass or fail. An assessment is made and sometimes a fact is declared. True or false.

Evidence is an important concept also in establishing a rationale or potential for action. Here there is no single criterion but multiple criteria: A training policy should be based on many factors, on evidence of many kinds. An education is good only if broad. A debate is argued in terms of several implications, with evidence presented not just to establish facts but to make an integrated case. A rationale needs to be pertinent to the action to be taken. The pieces of evidence should be interrelated.

Consider the rationale for assessing the quality of a training program. A program evaluator recognizes multiple goals, multiple expectations, multiple challenges, multiple standards—and then brings a body of evidence to light. All those pieces are put together in a synthesis of values, possibly resulting in a simple judgment but amplified in a reasoned, evidence-based argument. Such would be an evidence-based judgment of quality of a training program.

Whether practitioners or administrators, whether examiners or examinees, decision makers need facts *and* rationales for possible action. They need good evidence "to apply to their claims," as Anthony Kelly and Robert Yin (2007) put it. Evidence builds the confidence needed for good decision making.

> Facts are stubborn things; and whatever may be our wishes, our inclinations, or the dictates of our passions, they cannot alter the state of facts

and evidence. (John Adams, defense of the British soldiers on trial for the Boston Massacre, 1770, in *Bartlett's Familiar Quotations,* 14th edition, 1968, p. 462)

We might hypothesize that one could measure quality of evidence based on the quality of a decision made. A *process*-oriented evaluator might select a panel of decision makers to judge the quality of the decision made. Was the decision considered broadly enough? Was the reasoning sound? In other words, does the decision look good to other decision makers?

But an *outcomes*-oriented evaluator is hard pressed to find good evidence of the quality of decision making. Can the subsequent outcomes be attributed to that decision? Attribution of effects to that decision is usually problematic. And how can this decision be compared with any decision that was not made?

Milan Kundera examined the uncertainties of life in his 1984 book, *The Unbearable Lightness of Being.* Contemplating the choices—particularly the political and amatory choices—of Tomas, a surgeon in Prague during the Soviet occupation of Czechoslovakia, Kundera said:

> There are no means for testing which decision is better, because there is no basis for comparisons. We live everything as it comes, without warning, like an actor going on cold. . . . (p. 8)

> Any schoolboy can do experiments in the physics laboratory to test various scientific hypotheses. But man, because he has only one life to live, cannot conduct experiments to test whether to follow his compassion or not. (p. 34)

Kundera was saying, "People have little way to test the quality of their evidence."

7.2. UNBEARABLE LIGHTNESS OF EVIDENCE

In that book, Kundera's theme was that life is a collection of chance happenings, with every intention and choice vulnerable to overturn by circumstance and impulse. As he told it, everything in the world happens but once, and thus, although precious, human existence has little substance. We feel the unbearable lightness of being. Kundera described Tomas's first meeting Tereza, the traumatic love of his life:

Seven years earlier, a complex neurological case *happened* to have been discovered at the hospital in Tereza's town. They called in the chief surgeon of Tomas' hospital in Prague for consultation, but the chief surgeon *happened* to be suffering from sciatica, and because he could not move, he sent Tomas to the provincial hospital in his place.

The town had several hotels, but Tomas *happened* to be given a room in the one where Tereza was employed. He *happened* to have enough free time before his train left to stop at the hotel restaurant. Tereza *happened* to be on duty, and *happened* to be serving Tomas' table. It had taken six chance happenings to push Tomas towards Tereza. . . . so fortuitous a love, that would not have existed had it not been for the chief surgeon's sciatica. . . . (1984, p. 35)

In this vein, I ask you yourself to consider the evidence by which you, we, all of us, make our decisions—both large and small. However disguised, they are often fortuitous, personal, and situational. This is not a claim that we make our decisions capriciously. No, we factor in matters of great importance, but the weights we assign to different matters are subject to change, as we are burdened by new responsibility and enticed by new opportunity.

Many writers—Daniel Stufflebeam (1971) and Lee Cronbach (1974), for example—have set the main goal of social research as improvement in decision making. I do not. Decision options often change after we know the problem better. I prefer to think the main goal is improving understanding of how things work in their particular settings. That information may be useful for improving the thing studied, but aiming the research directly at improvement risks failing to examine adequately the complexity of the way it works.

Evidence of how well the thing is working is important. Sometimes the evidence should be oriented to outcomes. Often the most important evidence is the integrity of the ongoing transactions, the process, the way it is working.

The highest priority evidence of how the program works, be it local or national, can often best be found by studying the working processes. Production and efficiency and goal fulfillment and cost-effectiveness are outcomes that should not be ignored. And what the sponsors and staff and public want to know should not be ignored. But some of the main attention of qualitative research should be on how the people in charge are carrying out their responsibilities. And thus the evidence blueprinted in the research should include and often emphasize the evidence of performance of the managers[1] and service delivery people. To many observers, such personalized views of program quality will be weak, unstable, and transitory. We want so much to end up at a high level of confidence.

Evidence is an attribute of information, but it is also an attribute of persuasion. Evidence contributes to understanding and conviction. So do bias, and loyalty, and fashion, and culture. Evidence runs up against sharp competitors. And because it runs close to compassion and yearning, the evidence is unbearably light. To choose evidence that is more robust and probative is to change the question and to lower the priority of human judgment. Evidence should first be valid and relevant, and then, I argue, should be subordinate to judgment, crafted to user confidence, crafted to be persuasive.

Quality of evidence in social and educational fields is a personal matter as much as a statistical matter. It should not be thought that evidence-based research depends mainly on measurement. Evidence-based research should enable people to attain a deeper conviction of how the thing works and what to do about it. As it has ever been, personal confidence will lay the foundation for professional practice and national policy (Erickson, 2008).

7.3. TRIANGULATION

Qualitative researchers triangulate their evidence. That is, to get the meanings straight, to be more confident that the evidence is good, they develop various habits called "triangulation." The simplest, probably, is to "look again and again, several times." Signs at railroad crossings used to say, "Stop, Look, and Listen." Or, more important, look and listen from more than one vantage point. But triangulation also is to "member check": to ask the woman quoted if that is what she said. It is more than being careful; it is being skeptical that they were seen or heard right and checking further.

We used to say that triangulation is a form of confirmation and validation, but when we started giving more respect to multiple points of view, we saw that triangulation may be a form of differentiation

---

[1] Administrators often remove study of their own decisions from an external evaluation design, thinking that the staff is better equipped to gather this evidence.

(Flick, 2002). It may make us more confident that we have the meaning right, or it may make us more confident that we need to examine differences to see important multiple meanings. You might call it a win–win situation. If the additional checking confirms that we have seen it right, we win. If the additional checking does not confirm, it may mean that there are more meanings to unpack, another way of winning. If some clerks say, "the rules are unfair," but additional clerks say, "the rules are fair," it may be that there are two groups that need to be identified. It may be that the newly hired clerks or the clerks dealing with protests see it differently. With triangulation, our research can be improved either way.

What evidence needs triangulation? When are more data needed? Here are some statements that might be reported:

1. "The children all sat at tables."
2. "The village children sat at close-by tables; the immigrant children sat further away."
3. "Some immigrant children disregarded what the teacher asked them to do."

Here are four rules. Which applies to each of the three preceding statements?

a. If the description is trivial or beyond question, there is little need to triangulate.
b. If the description is relevant but debatable, there is some need to triangulate.
c. If the data are evidence for a main assertion, there is much need to triangulate.
d. If a statement is a person's interpretation, there is little need to triangulate the validity of the statement.

Here are some additional observations for the report.

4. "The teacher was irritated."
5. "Seating reflects institutional approval; sitting close to the teacher is a reward."
6. "The teacher said she was making children comfortable sitting by those they knew."

In most studies, Statements 1 and 6 would be seen as not needing thorough triangulation. If Statement 5 is important to the findings of the study, the interpretation needs more evidence than a single quotation. Several teachers could be asked. Evidence that hyperactive boys sometimes are seated close to the teacher might undercut the assertion. Triangulation sometimes helps the researcher recognize that the situation is more complex than first realized.

When knowledge is being constructed, no two observers construct it exactly the same. Complete confirmation is not possible, but views are partly agreed upon, partly not. When what is not agreed upon is unimportant, both triangulation outcomes are reported. What is agreed upon is reported as substantiated. When the "not agreed upon" is important, the different views should be looked at closely. Evidence that has been triangulated is more credible.

7.4. MIXED METHODS AND CONFIDENCE

One of the habits of qualitative researchers is using multiple methods. By that I mean using multiple ways (such as interviews and observation) of coming to better understand something within the study. But going further, "mixed methods" is using multiple methods interactively, not just using them somewhere in the same study. It means using them together consciously to study a single thing (e.g., an issue or relationship). Suppose the study is about how social work leadership works to get manageable caseloads in selected cities. It is likely that the qualitative researcher would dig into particular meanings and applications of this leadership using interviews, observations, review of documents, and perhaps adding life histories and dialogue analysis. Other topics might be investigated simultaneously, with or without mixing methods. If any topic is studied deliberatively, formally specifying the connection of the methods, the researcher is taking a mixed-methods approach (Creswell and Plano Clark, 2006, p. 1–7).

The primary reason for mixing the methods, of course, is to improve the quality of the evidence. One of the alternative leadership assertions may be that the senior leaders skirt around state regulations and emphasize agreements of understanding with individual families. It is probably not enough to find that this emphasis is clear in the mission statement of the offices and that the leaders were quoted to that effect in family orientation visits. Perhaps the researcher should inquire into the leaders' inquiry into reputations in the neighborhoods and into the annual review of social worker competence, even though that might take some extraordinary investigative reporting. Somehow we need multiple sources of evidence. You probably already know that good newspapers such as the *Washington Post* have required reporters to have several sources of evidence for a key finding and to use multiple methods to triangulate it. The *Post* also has its standards of evidence to maintain. And standards of writing.

> Challenges in writing up mixed methods inquiry remain considerable, as different methodological traditions involve quite different communication traditions that incorporate different technical criteria and norms, as well as different rhetorical and aesthetic criteria and norms for what makes a test compelling. (Greene, 2007)

We triangulate to increase the confidence that we will have in our evidence. Decision makers need confidence in the evidence, relying on both professional knowledge and research knowledge. Quantitative researchers have a great asset in inferential statistics in that they can quantify the confidence they have in rejecting a null hypothesis they have tested. They can announce that a finding is statistically significant at a certain level of confidence. Qualitative researchers have good ways of increasing the level of confidence in their findings but lack a numerical scale for stating that confidence. They do know they can increase confidence by triangulating with mixed methods, member checking, and using review panels (Creswell and Plano Clark, 2006, pp. 1–7; Johnson and Christensen, 2008, p. 439).

7.5. MEMBER CHECKING

Member checking is presenting a recording or draft copy of an observation or interview to the persons providing the information and asking for correction and comment. The researchers are seeking accuracy, their possible insensitivity, and new meanings. Are the facts right? Is the story complete? Will the draft be offensive to someone? Is it really more complex than that? If the person says the quotation or description is correct, that doesn't make it correct, but it helps to reduce the errors. And it helps greatly in protecting human subjects from being hurt. The researcher should persist in trying to get that confirmation or correction.

Before data gathering, the researcher should indicate to those to be observed and quoted an intention to member check. Unfortunately, often the "member" has little interest in it or has no time free to examine an excerpt. Obviously, the sooner the excerpt is presented, the greater the chances of a good member check. Waiting until one has lots of material from a data source person is seldom a good idea.

The material presented for member checking should not include either quotation or personal description of someone else who has not been member checked. That is difficult if the material is dialogue among persons. One should consider which bits of data are most critical and triangulate them first. And consider which person is most at risk and get that fixed up before showing it to others.

Member checking is a process vital to qualitative research, but it often works slowly. Not enough time has been allowed, or its importance is not apparent to the people studied. Often all that can be done is to give respondents good opportunity to respond, noting that reporting requirements or other deadlines necessitate this assistance by a date you specify.

7.6. REVIEW PANELS

It is an important strategy to have more than one person gather data, even though the budget and schedule do not encourage it. "Multiple eyes" is one of the most important triangulations. It is also important to have more than one person interpreting the most important data. Almost always there is a need for alternative explanations. Sometimes the extra help provides valuable confirmation, but usually the differences in view add depth to the perception. That's right. When observers disagree, the complexity often becomes clearer. And get this: It is seldom critical to resolve the differences of view as to which perception is more nearly correct. It simply is important to describe different interpretations of how things work.

In Section 3.5, dissertation research by Tom Seals (1985) was summarized. You may recall that his research question dealt with therapists' conceptions of gender issues in marital therapy. He compared four theoretical orientations: psychoanalytic, family systems, behavioral, and existential–experiential, hoping to make a contribution to counseling theory. He used four panels of therapists to obtain interpretations.

Seals recognized that therapists with different training and methods of therapy would see the counseling of Pete and Lisa differently. He expected to get different insights from each panel, possibly with contradiction. New issues would emerge midway and could alter subsequent data collection and the ways the research question would be interpreted. Seals predicted the study would mature in ways he could not anticipate. You may want to read Section 3.5 again to see illustration of the use of panels and "progressive focusing" (the topic we take up in the next section).

One might think that Seals could better have worked with all his panels at the same time and have arrived at the same findings. But his feeling from the beginning was that the complexities of the case and the ideas were almost overwhelming. He proceeded incrementally, confident that he could better keep track of what was going on and plan his next steps from better information. He quoted Matthew Miles and Michael Huberman (1984), saying that putting all conceptualization together at the beginning would be

> a serious mistake. It rules out the possibility of collecting new data to fill in the gaps, or to test new hypotheses which emerge during the analysis; it tends to reduce the production of what might be termed "rival hypotheses" that question the field-worker's assumptions and biases; and it makes analysis into a giant overwhelming task that both demotivates the researcher and reduces the quality of the work produced. (Miles and Huberman, 1984, p. 49)

Review panels, like member checking and using multiple observers, serve the purpose of triangulation.

In addition to multiple viewing and member checking, the researcher should get critical friends to review the progress at various times during the study. Brief progress reports can be circulated to a few people, sometimes the dissertation committee, with a request for a critical look. All this adds time to the research, time most researchers would prefer to use gathering more data. But sometimes improving the quality of the data is more important than increasing the volume.

It is important that the researcher seize unexpected opportunities to confirm and challenge the meanings of developing issues and relationships. But it is just as important to plan to (what mountain climbers call) "reconnoiter" the research design. Identifying and directing review panels is a greatly underused strategy. The panel can be large or small, formal or informal, and often should include persons with special experience or viewpoints, some of them different from the researcher's. Yes, one needs the support of admirers, but often the recognition of flaws and foolishness is more important.

7.7. PROGRESSIVE FOCUSING

Informal triangulation occurs as we carefully monitor progress of the research. The meanings of things need to be reconsidered all during the research. Let's examine the words of an early behaviorist, Ivan Pavlov (1936), advising his students:

> Gradualness! About this most important condition of fruitful scientific work, I never can speak without emotion. Gradualness, gradualness, gradualness. From the very beginning of your work, school yourself to severe gradualness in the accumulation of knowledge. (Bartlett, 1968, p. 818)

His advice should ring a bell: to school ourselves in deliberate accumulation of knowledge. That includes the growing knowledge of our research question, our methods, our sources of data, and whatever helps us with interpretation. Gradualness, care, skepticism, revision.

In our graduate schools, some professors urge students to come to understand a problem thoroughly before designing a study and before spending time in the field gathering data. But those are two different things. Often, spending time in the field is an essential part of designing a study. Yes, we want preliminary understanding of the research question. New researchers need extra time to get ready. There is too little time to learn the issues once in the field. We need to be prepared. We need to have practiced our methods. Still, the feeling among many qualitative researchers is that we often have been too committed to a plan, too fixated upon using certain variables, at the time we begin gathering data. We should be gradual, redesigning the study as we are doing it.

Sociologist Malcolm Parlett and historian David Hamilton (1977) spoke about three stages at which qualitative researchers (1) observe, (2) inquire further, and then (3) seek to explain. They said:

Obviously the three stages overlap and interrelate functionally. The transition from stage to stage, as the investigation unfolds, occurs as problem areas become progressively clarified and redefined. The course of the study cannot be charted in advance. Beginning with an extensive data base, the researchers systematically reduce the breadth of their enquiry to give more concentrated attention to the emerging issues. (p. 15)

This progressive focusing relies on what psychologist David Ausubel (1963) called "advance organizers." They are pivotal ideas, anticipations, frameworks for understanding what to do next. Everyone has advance organizers. They guide us—well or badly—as we try to figure something out. To try to make our plans more formal, we borrow from early anthropologist Bronislaw Malinowski (1922/1984) *foreshadowing questions*. At the outset of each study we may prepare a list of foreshadowing questions that need to be answered, topical (as opposed to methods) questions that help clarify the situation. Along the way we will abandon the unhelpful questions. We mean to reshape the questions to improve data gathering from one research site to the next.

In some studies, we will have a couple of years to focus "progressively" so as to improve the validity of our findings. My group had 2 years in our *Case Studies in Science Education* (Stake and Easley, 1978). In August 1975, the request for proposals (RFP) from the National Science Foundation included a long list of questions for the researchers to pursue. Those were their advance organizers. By July 1976, we had progressed to three foreshadowing questions:

1. How is science being taught in American schools?
2. What are the current conceptualizations of science in the courses?
3. What currently are the obstacles to science teaching?

By November the advance organizers had evolved to seven key issues:

1. *Budget cuts*: important at the sites, but later not seen to be an influence on teaching.
2. *Articulation*: the fitting together of courses from one year to the next; an emerging issue.
3. *Back to the basics*: opposition to a reform curriculum, anticipated and found important.

4. *Mastery learning*: not of interest to practitioners; of interest mostly to the researchers.
5. *Pedagogical theory versus practice*: anticipated big, turned out to be little at the sites.
6. *Teacher socialization*: increasingly a major reason for demise of the NSF-sponsored reform curriculum.
7. *Elitist teaching*: more attention to the able students, a stinging question; it was present but remained hidden; it was not of concern to most professionals in the field.

The list continued to be refined. Most of the original issues persisted, some faded, some new ones emerged.

The next May, I circulated an "early outline" of final chapter titles. Team member Terry Denny chided me for still seeing what I saw at the beginning, calling it "regressive focusing." Even after a year in the field, the picture was hazy. It was difficult to find a dominant structure of issues across sites. It was easy to argue that the issues identified for organizing the final report were, in fact, important findings at only half our sites. Our team could have included several other story lines. And other teams of researchers might have found the same data to tell of issues we missed.

It became increasingly apparent that, particularly with naturalistic studies, we are working through a merger of a research viewpoint (your viewpoint) and the activity in the field. There is a uniqueness to the way the researcher or research team sees things and a uniqueness to the sites. There are alternative stories to be told, even amid hopes for strong generalizations. We find that some audiences want researchers to bend every effort to present a report the same as other researchers would present, to tell the story that best represents the activity at the sites. But most audiences recognize the need for interpretation, personal insights. In the end, pretty much, we tell the story that seems most meaningful to ourselves.

The choice of "most meaningful" is subjective. We have numerous opportunities to check out views and patches with other researchers, with representatives of our audiences, with program staffs and others. Valuable as those negotiations are, particularly for correcting erroneous or offensive inclusions, they are weak grounds for progressive focusing. We rely greatly on intuition.

Progressive focusing is a slogan, a good slogan. It indicates our desire to keep observations and interpretations unfinished. But we sacrifice the increased power of instruments and protocols based on a fixed project design. Still, we can gain in relevance and timeliness. The changes in focus, "zooming in" on the target or shifting to another, remain a subjective choice, open to challenge or reinforcement by others. The interaction of researchers with their research sites remains something distinctive in each qualitative study.

Progressive focusing signals our commitment to gradualness, an effort to control presumption and invalidity. Perhaps we could say that this helps us salivate for high-quality research?

Does the message of this last section conflict with that of the previous sections of this chapter? Earlier we were talking about "bolstering judgment." And now we are talking about "moving on." We came to agree, I hope, that the research findings or assertions should be backed up by good evidence and that triangulation is the grand strategy for testing the quality of the evidence. One of the largest efforts to get triangulation is to use mixed methods, member checking, and panel review.

But then we talk of progressive focusing, where the meanings and data gathering and issues and prospective findings change throughout the study. Is it possible to get good evidence during the study if you do not know, toward the end of the study, what the research question is finally going to be? I hope you recognize that we have some explaining to do. How would you deal with this contradiction?

CHAPTER 8

Analysis and Synthesis
How Things Work

Research involves both analysis (the taking things apart) and synthesis (the putting things together). We gather data. We increase our experience. We look closely at the patches of collected data, the parts of our experience; that is, we analyze. And we put the parts together, often in different ways than before. We synthesize.[1]

Much qualitative research is based on the collection and interpretation of episodes. Episodes are held as personal knowledge more than as aggregated knowledge (Section 1.3). An episode has activities, sequence, place, people, and context. Some of the more useful-appearing episodes, the ones we think of as "patches," need to be studied, analyzed, their parts seen and seen again. We observe them, and we record other people's observations. We interpret them and seek other interpretations. We put things together and take them apart. As qualitative researchers, we

---

[1]In philosophy, a synthesis is the process of reconciling thesis and antithesis. Sometimes it is a useful idea for synthesis of qualitative research data if the data sort into two piles, those for and those against the research question or an assertion being considered. Assertions are important in qualitative research, but there are seldom just two sides to consider. The stories to be told, the understandings to be gained, have multiple dimensions. But the idea of presenting different views and showing favor for one more than the others is one of the good approaches. Mostly we will use the term *synthesis* just to mean putting the main separate patches together.

try to be especially sensitive to what are wholes, things that resist being taken apart, but still we analyze them. And sometimes we put the facts together into new wholes, into new interpretations, into a new patch.

We do much of this work intuitively. We use common sense. We follow certain routines. We triangulate. We follow the patterns of other researchers, as well as the patterns we ourselves used earlier. Sometimes we invent new ways to analyze and synthesize. Some of the work of our research is orderly—it could be more so—but deliberately inventive. Our work becomes centered on what we are finding, on our patches, but we come back again and again to the research question. We envision a report that will help other people understand things, too. We move from one understanding to another, with uncertainty, yet with a certain sense of composition. We are reshaping dialogues, portrayals, sometimes explanations, further insights into how something works.

8.1. TAKING APART AND PUTTING TOGETHER

Such a something for one researcher was haptic sensitivity. How does haptic sensitivity work, especially in art education? Haptic sensitivity is tactile, kinesthetic, bodily spatial awareness. In 2007, for her dissertation research in art education, You-Jin Lee of the University of Illinois chose to do a qualitative study of how such sensitivity may influence the making and teaching of art.

Her primary data were to come from observing four college classes: one in ceramics, one in graphic design, one in computer-based visual design, and one on the Japanese tea ceremony. She created the observation sheet shown in Figure 8.1 because she needed detail from each weekly classroom observation and she wanted to be reminded that most of her data were to be *interpretive* data, such as the actual words of the instructor and students at the very moment that there was reference to or evidence of the haptic. She also looked for *aggregative* data, such as showing how frequently someone referred to spatial relationships being felt in a bodily sense. Not only did she mark both front and back of the sheet while observing, but immediately afterward, she made further interpretations of what she had seen, heard, and perhaps felt.

Lee was working with an elusive concept. Beginning with her earliest preparation for the study, she needed to analyze this concept, haptic sensitivity. She sought definitions and wrote some of her own. She looked

Teacher code: Class code: Time: to:

Number of students: Artifact code: Observer:

Time/date of write-up: Extra copies filed under:

Lesson/Activities: Dialogue/Quotes:

Haptic elements:		Indications of quality made through:
Tactile	Movement (muscular–visceral)	Verbal articulation
Bodily awareness	Vibration	Written objectives
Balance	Space (physical/atmospheric)	Body language
Muscular–visceral	Rhythm	Questioning strategies
Temperature	Pain	Conversation
Moisture		Observation
Other nonvisual and nonauditory: Aroma, Taste		

Follow-up notes/conversations regarding observed action:

Extra features of the haptic:

Use of the haptic:	
Understanding	To understand materiality and affective aspects of media
Exploration	To discover new information and develop previously gained information
Inspiration	To use tactile experience as a source of ideas for and about arts
Concretization	To give a concrete form to an idea
Empathic viewing	To understand other people's emotion, feelings, situation, etc.
Perceptual sensibility	To use intuitive, visceral, nonaudiovisual features of understanding/making arts

Photographs/Artifacts collected: yes   no

Photographs/Artifacts needing to be collected: yes   no

Type of Document/Artifact:

FIGURE 8.1. Haptics Study Observation Form—You-Jin P. Lee, University of Illinois, August 2008 version. Reprinted with permission from You-Jin Lee.

for elements of such a sensitivity; that is, she analyzed the concept. Formally or informally, she created a concept map (Section 6.2). Early on, she tried to imagine what might be said in class that she could recognize as haptic awareness by teachers and students. She tried to imagine how the awareness would work to influence making art in different media. Ceramics was different from computerized spatial design. Maybe they would have little in common. She had done a pilot study, observing the meetings of instructors, looking further for traces of haptic sensitivity. Preanalysis. Presynthesis. At this point she constructed her observation sheet (Figure 8.1), including her idea of elements of haptic awareness, as shown in the box labeled "Haptic Elements."

The instructors in these four classes had an idea of what Lee was looking for and had assured her that they thought something of a haptic sensitivity was important in their classrooms. Lee anticipated that they might occasionally refer to bodily or tactile awareness but would not directly teach students to be aware of their awareness. The awareness might be what Michael Polanyi (1966) called "tacit knowledge":

> I shall reconsider human knowledge by starting from the fact that we can know more than we can tell. This fact seems obvious enough, but it is not easy to say exactly what it means. Take an example. We know a person's face, and can recognize it among a thousand, indeed among a million. Yet we usually cannot tell how we recognize a face we know. (p. 4)

Lee realized that what she was looking for might not be spoken directly. She needed to analyze further her early data. Even when her formal observations in the four classes began, she was still unsure, still analyzing what she might be looking for. Some might criticize her and her advisors for going ahead with so little explication, but in qualitative research we expect regeneration through progressive focusing (Section 7.7). Lee's research was pointed as much at how she was developing her methods of observing the haptic as at the data coming from those methods. Partly she was studying her own inquiry, a process that might become a finding in her dissertation.

In Chapter 11 we look in detail at the qualitative researcher emphasizing particularization over generalization. You-Jin Lee's four case studies were qualitative case studies. She was not seeking to represent other classes where art is taught and where haptic sensitivity might be important but to examine the relationships between the haptic and pedagogical phenomena in the places she directly observed. Later, she and her readers would refine the study of those relationships and might use them in the design of instruction and modification of visual art curriculum theory. Inside her study, Lee gave some thought to generalization, but her primary intent was on analyzing and understanding particular episodes. (Lee's study continued beyond the completion of my book.) This I predict:

> From day to day, upon encountering a particularly pertinent observation, Lee will describe individual episodes for *microanalysis*, seeking the meaning of each instance. Her memory, her audio recording, her notes on the observation guide, and the occasional interview write-up will help her reconstruct and analyze and write up the episode, the patch. Later in the study, she will find patches that fit together, a synthesis. The guide sheets and episode descriptions will be sorted according to subissues and elements of haptic awareness. She will examine the clusters separately, interpreting them in terms of her issues and research question, making *issue commentaries* (more patches). Her analysis will continue as aggregation of these commentaries during the progress of the study. Toward the end of data gathering, she will start drafting *chapters* that report the best of these episodes, analyses, and commentaries. She will go through them a number of times, triangulating, getting help from reviewers, refining the interpretations and generating newly perceived counterpositions. If this sounds formulaic, let me assure you as I did her that if the thinking and recording have been done well, the dissertation half writes itself.

Research is not only aimed at the substantive assertions to be produced but is also about coming to understand your own particular inquiry better (Becker, 1998). What I mean to say is that, during research, analysis and synthesis are ongoing, interactive, habituated inquiry processes. In qualitative research, analysis is seldom a formal set of calculations at a certain phase between data gathering and interpretation. Analysis and synthesis continue from the beginning of interest in the topic and continue still into the hours at the keyboard writing up the final report.

8.2. WORKING WITH PATCHES

The best observations made by You-Jin Lee can be thought of as patches, to be sorted in different ways, to be synthesized with photo patches and quotation patches and rumination patches. Different patterns emerge. In Figure 8.2 you can see a small collection of patches from You-Jin's study.

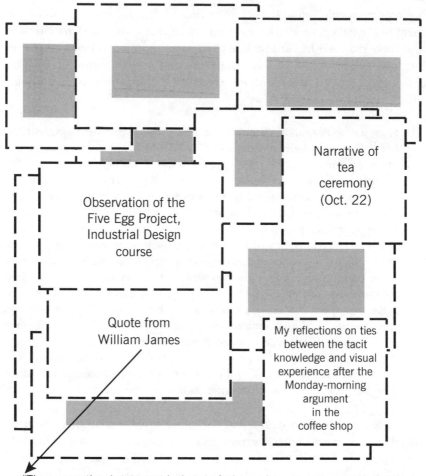

Narrative of
tea
ceremony
(Oct. 22)

Observation of the
Five Egg Project,
Industrial Design
course

Quote from
William James

My reflections on ties
between the tacit
knowledge and visual
experience after the
Monday-morning
argument
in the
coffee shop

"The more rational statement is that we feel sorry because we cry, angry because
we strike, afraid because we tremble, and not that we cry, strike, or tremble
because we are sorry, angry, or fearful, as the case may be. Without the bodily
states following on the perception, the latter would be purely cognitive in form, pale
colorless, destitute of emotional warmth."

FIGURE 8.2. Patches to work into You-Jin Lee's final report.

Using electronic copies or photocopies, Lee's patches would be stored for each of her four classrooms, stored also according to the issues, stored also according to the elements of the haptic, probably in some other ways as well. Gradually she would rearrange these pieces as the study moves along and increasingly sense how to organize the final report. We talk about that synthesis in Section 8.3.

I want to show you a long patch. I do not have a good example from Lee's study. I will show you a complex story patch from a Chicago elementary school, illustrating key issues. It describes a bubble gum experiment (Box 8.1). It came from research on the professional development being provided by the Chicago Teachers Academy for Mathematics and Science (Stake, 2000). Look for whether or not, as you see it, this long patch would be useful in telling how the Academy's professional development worked.

This was a story about people trying to find how something worked. How did the brands of bubble gum compare? How did the experiment work? How did this mathematics teaching work amid ethical disturbance? The story tells how they worked and did not work in Miss Grogan's classroom. We talk more about stories in Chapter 10.

The description of the activity in Grogan's room illustrates a number of things we are trying to accomplish in qualitative research. We try to observe and record closely so that we can describe it in ways the reader can experience it, having the feeling of being alongside the observer. The passing of the day, the permanence of the physical space, the nearness of the rest of the school and neighborhood are signals: the wind, the sirens, someone wearing boots walking by the door. What does this have to do with how things work? Remember the epistemological idea: The meanings of the phenomena are influenced by even barely observable happenings. The teacher has an explanation ready if the principal inquires about the noise. Miss Grogan may not want to tell Miss Jackson her calculation didn't work. The meanings of a happenstance mathematics lesson reach out into the complexities of professional development, social status, parental expectations of education—to countless complexities. These complexities seldom get identified in the research question or the research plan. They become recognized by the roaming mind of the researcher and put into a patch for reflection, review, and possible placement in the final report.

(text resumes on p. 149)

BOX 8.1. The Bubble Gum Experiment

On the last Friday in May, Miss Grogan announced that for the mathematics lesson, they would do research on bubble gum. She had been counting out pieces earlier, and several children had stretched to see what she was doing. After they returned from computer class, she quieted them.

1:07: "Clear your desks, except for your notebook." It becomes quiet, each at his/her own place. Grogan points to five stations around the room, each with a poster identifying a bubble gum brand name and a small supply of gum.

"Okay. Just after lunch I told you we would do some research on bubble gum and drawing some graphs. What rules for the research did I mention?" (Silence, but happy anticipation that something good is going to happen.) "We are going to make graphs of bubble size and elasticity."

"There are different kinds of bubble gum, and we don't know if they are equally good at making bubbles. Each of you will make a bubble with each of five brands and, using plastic dividers, a teammate will measure the diameter." (She has placed meter sticks and calipers at each station.) "Each of you should record the measurements in your journals and on the posted sheet. Then you will take the gum, pull it into a string, and see how far you can stretch it, measuring the length with a meter stick.

"As soon as you have made both measurements, wrap that piece of gum in its wrapper and put it in the paper cup. Do not put gum anywhere except in the cup at the station. If you get it on the floor, you *must* clean it up. We don't want bubble gum on the floor or under the chairs." (Carlos claims there is gum stuck under *her* desk.) She repeats, "Put the used gum in the cups."

"Listen up. Another rule is: When chewing, it's only one stick. I trust you not to take any extra. The experiment will only work if you chew one piece. If you wad up your mouth with gum, the experiment won't work. [*pause*] We might have a problem if someone has a big mouth. Some people may be able to blow better than others." [*laughter*]

"Let's be serious about this. We don't want Mrs. Bravo coming in and think we are goofing off. But she will understand that an experiment is important."

1:25: "We need five teams, three or four, possibly five, persons to a team. Each team is in charge of the record for one brand of gum. Is it time to break into groups? [pause] Now, divide yourselves into groups."

(cont.)

BOX 8.1. *(cont.)*

There is a fluttering about. Four of the more intellectually mature gather at one table, then a second group forms. Most others stay at their seats, waiting to see how things shape up—then one by one they approach and sit down with a pair or threesome. No one approaches an existing foursome. There are now five groups of four and three kids left over; now Carlos joins the three to make a group. A couple of groups continue to reorganize, finally leaving two girls without a bubble gum station. They don't seem to mind, chatting together.

"Desks clear except for notebooks and pencils. In your journal, write the names of the people in your group." (Each person keeps their own notebook.) "Put down your own name too." Now two boys switch groups, leaving all groups but one with a single gender.

"Next, write down the names of the bubble gum, leaving space for each. Okay, do we need to know if all the gum pieces are of equal size? [A couple of hesitant yeses.] Let's find out and enter each size in your journal."

1. Bazooka. "How many grams in each stick, Monica?" She reads the label: "Five grams per stick." "Write it."
2. Bubble Yum. "Alejandro, how much in each Bubble Yum stick?" "Five grams."

[All are writing, though Alfonso has to be stared down to get him started.]

3. Carefree Bubble Gum. "Veronica, how much in each stick?" "Two point five grams."
4. Bubblicious. "Maria, how much in each stick" "Eight grams."
5. Extra Bubble Gum, Sugar Free. "Claudio, how big is each stick?" "Two point seven grams."

"Now do your bubbles and record your results. First diameter, then elasticity. Record your results at each station. [Murmuring] David, if you tattle, that will get you in trouble too."

1:45: All are busy chewing gum, more or less quietly. Miss Grogan reminds them they have to record other people's results, that they are doing an experiment in mathematics. Omar gently affixes the plastic tips to measure David's bubble. Touching Anna's pink sphere, Angela reads the angle at 32 degrees. Amelia objects, saying that the others

(cont.)

BOX 8.1. *(cont.)*

are measuring in centimeters. Now they decide to see if Anna can get a larger bubble.

Claudio stretches his gum to 2 meters but records it as 2 inches. Roberto's pursuit of stretch threatens to get out of hand. Sammy has stretched his over 10 feet. It is not possible to keep the strand off the floor. Someone tells Grogan. She again says to stop tattling. "The next time I hear tattling, I'm going to. . . . " As to elasticity, we seem close to being in trouble. There is no place to go without crossing someone's strand. But Grogan has a smile on her face and a camera 'round her neck.

"Make sure you have recorded both length and bubble size on the paper. Time is up for your first readings. You should have both your recordings for the first piece of gum. Change stations and do it over again."

THE CRISIS

Then, "Stop! Everyone, stop! The Bubblicious is all gone! It needs to be returned. Only four people had taken a piece. The box was full. Sit down. You blew it." (No pun acknowledged; Grogan is shouting in anger.)

Pointing to a stick of gum, Gabriel says, "There is Bubblicious on my desk." As is often the case, he is ignored. Most are still talking to each other. Grogan doesn't speak for what seems a minute. Then, "There had to be at least 10 or 15 there. I said that the only way this experiment would work was if we worked as a team. If we have extra, then we can hand them out. Somebody abused this. When things get abused, they get taken away. Carlos? Anybody? I am very disappointed. This is the first time something like this has happened. Nobody is going to confess or return it? [Silence.] All right."

She goes out of the room (we two observers follow). Then she returns. "Enough. Return to your seats. We are going to take the numbers we have and calculate the results." (Another long delay as the kids take their seats.) "Okay, we are going to add up the numbers and get the average, the mean, M-E-A-N, mean. Here they are in centimeters, write them down: 3.1, 2.6, 4.2, 3.5, 3.0, 2.9, 4.0, 3.8, 2.6, 3.5, and 3.1. Add those numbers up. [Long pause.] "After you finish adding those

(cont.)

BOX 8.1. *(cont.)*

numbers, count how many scores there are." (She counts.) "There are 11 scores. You are going to divide your total by 11." (A strained minute goes by.)

Miss Grogan bends over individuals at length, making terse comments. Some of the students seem to be struggling. Others sit quietly looking around. Grogan suggests they check their work. Now, all heads are down. There has been no reminder of the purpose for calculating this average.

2:15: "You may want to double-check it." This takes a very long time. "Double-check your answers." (It's as if she has just found a mistake. The decimals seem to invite mistakes.) "Be sure you have lined your numbers up right. Juan, are you done? What do you do with your total after you get it?" Carlos says, "I messed up, I believe."

It becomes apparent that Grogan does not intend to do anything with the means today. She says, "Count to yourselves. Everybody is messing each other up. Maybe if I was in a better mood, I would let you use calculators. But you messed that up too." She continues to go about the room, looking at calculations, making quiet suggestions. Chastising David, she says, "First of all, you don't do math with a pen."

Then, "David, go get water for the boards. There shouldn't be any talking. [Pause] Okay, stop what you are doing. Put your names on your worksheets. Without a sound, Alejandro. Then I want everyone's attention." She is glaring at Alejandro.

"What would you rather have done, the bubble gum experiment or this? Who would rather do the worksheet?" Only Carlos raises his hand. "Veronica asked me if she could use a calculator. At another time, I might have said, 'Okay,' but you need to be able to do this in your head. On a test you sometimes cannot use a calculator. Any comments on what happened this afternoon?" (No answer, but she waits.) Angela says, "You are mad." Looking around the class, "I would be a lot less mad if you had been honest. It takes a lot less to confess than to do this.

"You have 2 weeks of school left after today. We can go back to worksheets and reading the book. I suggest that, over the weekend, you decide whether or not we should give the class a second chance. I am really hurt. I don't go buying 16 packs of gum just to embarrass myself. Maybe I shouldn't take a chance having Mrs. Bravo come in seeing you chewing bubble gum. One thing nice about it, there were no wrappers

(cont.)

BOX 8.1. *(cont.)*

on the floor. So, Monday we will discuss it. And maybe I will give you a second chance."

2:30: "If you want to bring it up anonymously, we can do it. You will have to prove to me that I can trust the class. As I said, this is the first time this has happened in this class. It is up to you. You may get your stuff ready to go home."

What happened during this mathematics class illustrated Miss Grogan's attachment to the children, her concern about their social development, and her desire to use the kinds of mathematics activities promoted by the Academy. She was nearing the end of the year, and it was going to be a difficult separation for her as well as the children. She had formed personal attachments to each of them, and they for her. Hour after hour on most days went by without an expression of disrespect. Frequently she would yell "One," then "Two," then "Two and a half" to get things quiet and she would sometimes stare long and hard at someone not complying with her immediate expectation, but they seldom got close to a crisis. On this day, in Grogan's eyes, they had crossed the line.

Like the high majority of teachers, new and experienced, Miss Grogan appeared here to sacrifice a good learning opportunity for a social development opportunity. She could have postponed the resolution of the lost gum, carrying on the experiment with the remaining four brands. Having five brands was not critical to the activity. But it was important for her to show that trust had been breached, that theft and possibly collusion should not be treated lightly. This choice between academic learning opportunity and social ethics opportunity is not uncommon in elementary schools everywhere but is seldom discussed. It is the teacher's sense of propriety that decides, and the choice made by Miss Grogan would be supported regularly by other teachers and parents. When asked about it, a number of children in Academy-affiliated schools also have expressed support for maintaining decorum and punishing misbehavior, even at the cost of good learning activities.

Miss Grogan was deeply disappointed not only with her children but with the failure to complete the graphing experiment. She recognized in retrospect that looking at elasticity as well as bubble size was more than time would allow. If all had gone well, she would not have had time that day for each child to finish a bar graph and to discuss its meanings, asking whether such things as gum weight and mouth size might have distorted the results. She was used to activities that contin-

(cont.)

BOX 8.1. *(cont.)*

ued beyond a single day, but, as with other teachers we have observed, not every interrupted project gets resumed. Grogan was enthused about having such standards-based and motivating activities, and appreciated the mathematical explanations she got from the Academy, and the curtailing of this one started her weekend on a very bad note.

CONTINUATION

It is the following Tuesday. "Okay! Does everyone have a calculator? Math notebooks should be open to the section of the page where we were recording those numbers that you were adding and subtracting. What I would like to do is to get the other. . . . One! Two! Monica! I am going to give you the opportunity to check the answers you got yesterday." She hands out hand calculators to each student.

Bubble Yum   20, 10, 11, 7.5, 7.5, 7.5, 14.5, 14.5, 8.5, 18.5, 2

Extra   5.3, 3, 2.7, 4, 4, 4, 6.6, 7.9, 7.5, 7.7, 11.3, 6, 6.5, 3, 3

Bubblicious 5.5, 9, 10, 9, 4, 7, 8, 12, 8.5, 12, 23, 14, 7.7

Bazooka   10, 14, 11, 5, 11, 11, 2.5, 7, 7, 19

Carefree   5, 6, 7, 6, 4, 5, 5, 7, 5, 3, 2, 7, 8, 6, 8

"Yesterday you calculated the averages for the first three bubble gums. Now, you need to do the last two." All are quickly at work, most using hand calculators. David asks for help. "Which are the whole numbers?" He points to them. Roberto asks about dividing on the calculator.

"Omar, are you done with all five?" She goes back to the board and makes the commas between all numbers more legible. There is some consternation at one table about the contents of a water bottle, a breakout of laughter. "Angela!"

Grogan's red hair is even more a lion's mane today. She tells me that things went well yesterday. She had handed a piece of each brand of gum, a sack to each student, had told them they had just 10 minutes to make their measurements.

At 12:35 she says, "Okay, stop. [Pause] Okay, what was your average for Bazooka? Lisa? She says, "9.75." "What did you get for Care-

(cont.)

BOX 8.1. *(cont.)*

free, Anna? What did you get when you divided?" "I didn't divide it." "Why didn't you?" [Glare] Someone says, "Carefree: 5.6."

"What about Bubble Yum? I only have four who have answers?" She stands by the table that works the least. "David, are you done?" "No." "Then why are you talking? Anna, what did you get?" Anna looks distressed. When Grogan walks away, Anna bites her nails. Her tablemates look away. Grogan shows she is anxious to have each do the work. Right now there is diligence but she is not getting real productivity. There is a low level of interest in the problem. It has become work. The gum has lost its flavor.

"So the average for Bubble Yum is what? Monica?" [No answer] "Juan?" "I don't have the answer." "Then why are you looking all over the place? . . . Esperanza, what did you get? "11.0." Someone else says, "I got 11.9." "How many got 11.9? . . . Five. Sammy, what did you get? Everybody, stop what you are doing. Clear your calculator. We are going to do this together."

Simultaneously they enter the numbers as Grogan reads them off. Looking at her calculator, she says, "You should have 121.5. Press divide. Hey! We have 11 numbers. So we are going to divide by 11. So 11.0 is correct. If you didn't get that, you didn't add right. You can easily make an error. The calculator cannot do it right if you do not put the decimals in right."

"Yesterday we got 12.0." "Oh, I made an error. Sorry. Well, I used Juan's notes. Everybody, clear your calculator. We are going to do Extra. Everybody clear." Once again she reads the numbers aloud and they enter them into their calculators, running awry midway and having to start over.

"What's the total?" "103." "How many got 103? [Pause] Then we divide by [she counts] by 18. 5.72. [a bit of giggling] Hey, this is not funny. We have a lot of work to do. Angela, do you have it written down? Let's just stick with what we did together. 103 divided by 18 gives you 5.7. Extra is 5.7."

The same procedure is followed for Bubblicious. Most get 136 for the total and dividing by 14, the modal response is 9.7. Is that right? Grogan is impatient because so many are not getting the same sum. And the routine is followed for Bazooka and Carefree.

On the blackboard at the back of the room is a large rose sketched in chalk. The words underneath are: "Miss Grogan is the best."

(cont.)

BOX 8.1. *(cont.)*

AVERAGES

"Does everyone have the average?" "Yes." "This is not the only average. There are three of them. The names of the three averages are mean, median, and mode. Mean. Median. Mode." She writes the three words on the board. "The mean is what you just did. The second average is the median. It has an 'n' at the end. To find the median, I want to show you a trick Miss Jackson taught me."

The numbers for Bazooka gum are still on the board. Grogan crossed off the 10 at the left end of the row and the 19 at the right end. She repeated that, left and right, until four measurements were crossed off on each end, leaving only the middle two 11s not crossed off. She says, "These 11s are the same, so the median is 11." She had failed to put the measurements in order of increasing value. She had indicated that the median is the middle number in a row of unsequenced data.

She goes on to the mode. She identifies the mode as the number that occurs most frequently in a set of data. "It's whatever score comes out the most. So for Bazooka, 11 comes up the most. What does median mean? Median, Anna? What is the median? I just told you?" Grogan goes on to tell about the median on a highway.

"What is the mode?" Angela says, "The number that shows up the most . . . " "Give me the mode of Bubble Yum." "7.5 is the mode for Bubble Yum." "What is the mode for Extra, Carlos? There are three 4s, only two 7s. What about Bubblicious?"

Listen, I am going to give you back the worksheet you had on Friday. Tomorrow we are going to graph this information. Do not tear it out of the notebook. What are you going to do, Monica?" "Math." "What is there to do for math?" "The worksheets."

On Monday of the following week, I return to Audubon. In the hallway, I notice a colorful and large new poster with the question, "Which bubble gum makes the largest bubbles?" The answer displayed is "Bubblicious." About a dozen 8½ × 11 graphs are displayed, each showing five monotonic traces, color coded as shown in its legend for the five brands of gum. The graph Harry did is shown in Figure 8.3.

The 11 or so other graphed functions looked pretty much the same as Harry's, but not exactly. Harry and the other students had numbered the ordinate from 1 to 34 and the abscissa from 1 to 35 but nothing further to identify the two variables. For Harry's, I presumed that the

(cont.)

BOX 8.1. *(cont.)*

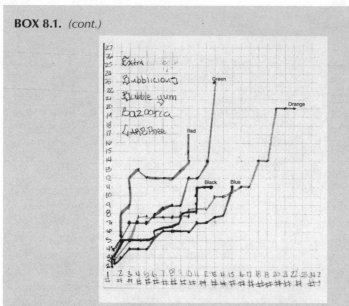

FIGURE 8.3. Five-color line drawing submitted by Harry in his report.

baseline numbers represented students, with 13 students having provided Bubblicious measurements, and that the vertical measure was bubble size in centimeters. Grogan confirmed that later. I asked her also if it was because the largest of all bubbles recorded had come from Bubblicious, one of 23 centimeters diameter, that it was declared the winner. Grogan said, "No," that the conclusion about biggest bubbles was made before the graphing had been done. The five means had been compared, and Bubblicious had the largest mean. So, although I did not witness that fourth class period, the students apparently had compared average sizes for the five brands and named the winner, completing the experiment originally planned.

The experiment had begun in enthusiasm, had moved through trauma, had become pretty much a follow-the-rules routine, had included teaching of a misunderstanding, and had ended with a product that needed further questioning, which it did not get. It was apparent that Grogan did not understand all the mathematics involved in the exercise and asked only Miss Jackson for help. I have described this

(cont.)

BOX 8.1. *(cont.)*

episode to several mathematics educators, and they were considerably dismayed. My own analysis was that the students had learned more than they had mislearned, that in no way had they been hurt.

What I saw them getting from the several math periods was the sense of a science or engineering study. It required thinking about comparison, about causation, and about measurement, e.g., representing size and elasticity with numbers. They were supposed to learn something about central tendency of a distribution, but they learned very little. They may have mislearned something about the median, but since they dealt with the concept of middleness so briefly, their miscalculation probably was of little consequence. They had an experience of trying to solve a problem, to do an experiment, to arrive at an answer to an interesting question using their mathematical skills. It was not a demonstration. They did the thinking. The teaching was not the success it might have been, but it provided a sustained opportunity to carry out an experiment.

With a succession of graduate students, I had been evaluating the professional development activities of the Academy for 5 years. Each year we prepared a report, indicating our observations of the staff work and the work of participating teachers. I had visited Miss Grogan's classroom several times before this multiday math project. I did not expect it to be a story that I would want to publish in detail, but I did and am doing so again here.

The Academy trainers had encouraged teachers to do projects and even to consider teaching about experiments. Somewhere they had included a lesson for the teachers on action research and another on indicators of central tendency. I did not follow up with questions to Grogan as to how she had planned this project because I felt she was embarrassed both by the theft of gum and by the error in calculating the median.

I described a bit of the context here and in other descriptions of Grogan's professional activity: her participation in staff development and admiration for the Academy, her Hispanic neighborhood, the features of the school, including its hallway exhibits and its vigorous teaching of the arts. I tried to think of how the context was influencing her teaching: the support of other teachers and parents, the aspirations of the principal, the involvement of the Chicago schools in more than 10 years of "school reform." They were potential parts of the bubble gum story, but the story already was long. For my Academy readers, it seemed not important to explain further why things worked or did not work in this project. As a qualitative researcher, I wanted to portray the episode in ways that the Academy staff and others could use in their work.

This story was, and so yours will be, enhanced by attention to the persons: Grogan's theatricality, Sammy's impetuousness, Gabriel's being ignored. It was enhanced by having a deep theme: Is getting things right, morally and academically, more important than staying immersed in a conceptual problem-solving situation? It raised the question of whether or not a visiting researcher who knows how to calculate the median should intervene to assist in the teaching. Many such questions arise spontaneously, some anticipated a little and some requiring impulsive decisions as to how the study will be useful.

This patch was used as one of three parts of the Year 2000 annual report of the evaluation of the Chicago Teachers Academy. It contains a chronological account of happenings in the classroom, a rich description (but without connection to a scientific theory, not a thick description) of the mathematics being taught, and some interpretation of the connection with teacher continuing education. We should connect with Chapter 2 and talk more about interpretation. We are moving toward the last third of this book and need to focus on our assertions and assembling the final report.

8.3. INTERPRETATION AND SORTING

Telling how it works is both description and interpretation. Sorting is a part of interpretation. In Chapter 2 we observed that qualitative research is sometimes called interpretive research. So, too, are historical and philosophical research. Quantitative research is interpretive, too, but much less so depending on what the researcher interprets experientially. Frequently using themselves as their instruments, qualitative researchers find much meaning coming from their own experience, as well as experience with people they interview, and as learned about from documents.

In Chapter 1 we distinguished between macroresearch and microresearch. The sizes differ—the worldly versus the local—but also the data differ. The analyses are different, and the interpretations are of a different kind. Macroresearch regularly deals with large bodies of data from lots of places, but the uniqueness of each of those places washes out in the analysis and interpretation. So the local context is unimportant, treated as "error variance." With quantitative inquiry, such differences are seen as worth paying attention to only if those differences can be aggregated, such as differences based on race or time of the year built into the design.

Coding (classifying, sorting) is a common feature of microresearch and all qualitative analysis and synthesis. Coding is sorting all data sets according to topics, themes, and issues important to the study. Coding is for interpretation and storage more than for organizing the final report. It can be structured by the research question, by a concept map, and by the clusters of patches developing. It can start early or be held back until most of the data are collected. The code categories are progressively focused, changing as the research question takes on new meanings and as the fieldwork turns up new stories and relationships. But those changes mean that data already coded may have to be recoded. Coding classifies all data. The data most worth including in the final report are identified as patches. The April boxes will usually look like the coding plan. Some advice about coding and storage is presented in Box 8.2.

Qualitative microresearch pays attention to lots of local situations, especially situations that can be experienced by the researcher. The effects of "zero tolerance leadership," for example, may range widely depending on hostilities held by the staff, community leaders, and the state legislature. The individual episodes of that leadership will be at the center of the interpretation. Often, the qualitative researcher makes much of his or her interpretations from personal experience with the people studied. The data would be different, the analysis and the grounds for interpretation would be different from those collected from large-scale surveys. In the qualitative report, fewer would be the tables, more would be the dialogues and vignettes. Often stories are told in a way that helps readers make their own interpretations. We talk more about synthesis in Chapter 11.

A graphic plan that can facilitate interpretation (perhaps I should have told you about it earlier) is a chart for preparing assembly of the final report or dissertation. I encourage researchers to start this plan in the early stages of the study, maybe not too long after obtaining institutional review board approval. The chart is shown as Figure 8.4.

BOX 8.2. Data Storage Tips

1. Keep a personal research log partly as a backup to data storage. Make note of patches.
2. Link your document storage to data gathering and writing. Many of the main documents are what you create, including designs, sketches, notes, tallies, photos, analyses, and interpretations.
3. Early on, make a mock-up of the final report, with tentative page allocation. Do not start assigning patches to places in the report. If you're working in a team, writing tasks should be assigned to the other members, too.
4. The writer of a topic or section should be in charge of document storage for that topic.
5. Too few files and too many files are both a mistake. Have a file at least for each issue, activity site, data source (person), pattern, context, box, and section of the final report.
6. You may want to prepare a statement of just-gathered data for the first draft of the report. You should provide a copy of those statements to other team members, if any. (Some progress on report writing should occur almost every day.)
7. Researchers accustomed to working with computer storage of ongoing research can make their main files electronic. Others should make their main files paper files.
8. Major data records should be routinely duplicated and stored in more than one file.
9. Records and statements needing discussion (with other team members or research supporters) should be marked, such as clipped with a red star. Regularly scheduled data discussions are desirable for clarification and triangulation.
10. Because of the press of time, audio- and videotapes should be used and transcribed only when it is clear that they are vital to the final report.
11. Found documents should be numbered and stored and brief information about them should be placed in appropriate files.
12. Your memory will be an important storage for writing the final report. One way to make memory more reliable is to keep a good log, including names, telephone numbers, addresses, dates and times, musings.

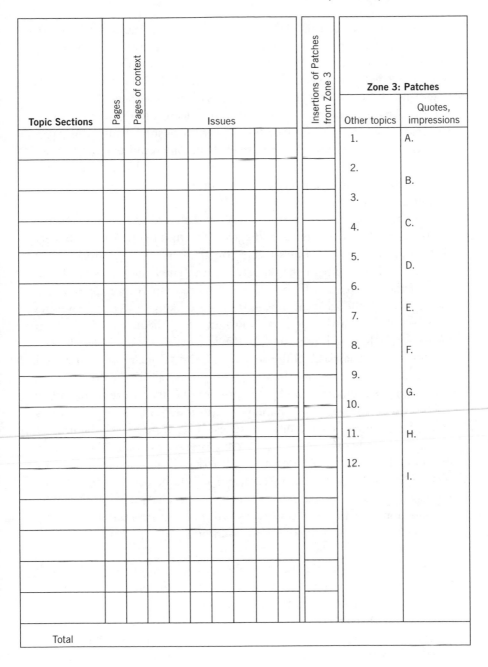

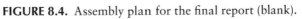

FIGURE 8.4. Assembly plan for the final report (blank).

One purpose for this plan (Figure 8.4) is (at an early date) to estimate and allocate pages to be used in the report. (A filled-in copy of the form is in Figure 11.3.) Of course one does not know how many pages will be needed. But some things are known: If the report is too short, it will not be respected; if too long, it will be little read. Some organizations have a standard report format. Electronic reporting can be less restrictive of page use. We all have report deadlines and 200 pages sometimes take less time to write than 100. Paper and postage are not free. Considering a dissertation, let's estimate the total at 180 pages, not including bibliography and appendices—more or less the median for our disciplines of study.

On the blank chart of Figure 8.4, you should write "180" below the boxes in the column headed "Pages." The first big task is to allocate those 180 pages to the topics (boxes or chapters). If you already have an outline of the study or the report, you can enter the topics on the 16 lines of the left column. If you have lots more than 16, for the moment merge some of the adjacent topics. If you are likely to use conventional chapter titles for a dissertation, you can enter them, something like: "Abstract," "Research Question," "Review of Literature," "Methods," "Fieldwork," "Analysis," "Interpretation," and "Conclusions." (I do not like headings that fail to tell anything substantive about the dissertation, but the choice is up to you and your superiors.) Chances are there will be 5–10 chapters. Some of the chapters need subdivision. In You-Jin Lee's study, for example, she might want to use a separate row on Figure 8.4 under the "Fieldwork" chapter for each of her four sites. In the example in Figure 11.3, the topic titles more clearly indicate the content of the section. The cells of the "Pages" column should be penciled in with the number of pages you estimate are needed and allowable. Soon it may become apparent that some sections will need to be shortened, partly because it is not desirable to tell all you know. Your pencil should have an eraser.

On to the "Pages of context" column: In a qualitative study, it will be important to allocate some extensive writing to context, to the organizational, community, political, economic, and historical settings for this research. Even though it is too early, it is good to start to get an idea of what sections you are going to tell about these. You might have "Contexts" as a main topic, but even so, some description of context is likely to be needed elsewhere. Indicate the number of pages out of those you inserted in the pages column that you would use for describing contexts. It is not a bad idea to note (in really small print) which contexts you are talking about in that row. Estimate the pages and pages of context for each of your topics rows.

That is enough page allocation. From here on we are just going to place stuff in topic rows. The next six columns are for big themes or issues that run through the report. One theme in Lee's haptic final report may be about feeling the materials that will be touched by hand: the clay, the computer printouts, the china teacups. If this happens to be the third of her issues (thus in the fifth of the narrower columns), she would check the rows (the main topic places) where she would expect to give more than a mention to these materials. She is not going to deal with "touched by hand" in all 16 topical spaces. If the issue were that prominent, she would use one of her main topic rows for it. (Remember that there is another example in Figure 11.3.)

Using this assembly plan for the first time, you may have little idea of what to put where. But doing it can be helpful. You need to make guesses as to where ideas may go. You will change pages and locations. Increasingly, you will realize how little space there will be. And this should help you think about how to spend your time in gathering data. There are likely to be good opportunities for which, if you pursue them, you would use far too many pages, giving those matters too much emphasis in the report. You need to discipline yourself to resist spending another day at a site for which you already have more data than you can report. Too many data of one kind, even really good data, throw a report out of balance. Yes, the next datum to be gathered might make it better, and on and on, but you have a life to live beyond doing this report.

The tenth and final blocked column is for placement of patches, important items that will be included only in one place, some dialogues, perhaps some impressions and quotes. Important but not to be presented several times. One such patch was that good quote by William James. Lee might have written it on Line M in the quotes column; if she decides to put it in Main Topic 2, she would insert the letter M in the Insertions of Patches column on the second horizontal row. All the "to-mention-once" topics and quotes will be identified with a main topic somewhere there in the six narrow columns. This is partly to help avoid using something unintentionally in more than one place.

The value of this assembly plan is partly in helping you get an early sense of the final report and to help you keep track of your patches.[2] The plan can be changed, and you can schedule a periodic reworking of the planner to include new and changed things that come up.

Analysis is the search for both elements and associations. Figure 8.1 includes a list of elements. The final report of research also is a form of synthesis, putting it all together. There are few recipes for analysis and synthesis. They are intuitive processes, but forms can help. But also, they can divert you from more important tasks, like straightening the books on your shelf.

Earlier experiences and the experience of doing the research are structures for synthesis. A good research design, a good review of the literature, good storage of data, all contribute to saying how and what you have to say about how a thing works. Some of us just sit down and start writing. But in a short while we open files of patches and pull volumes off the shelf. We do not ignore how others have described the working. It is plagiarism if you copy the assertions another researcher has published, but it is good sense to follow the writing process of a more experienced researcher. As they once said on short-wave radio, "Do you copy?"

---

[2] Patches often tell the unexpected. They tumble from a file or recollection, unsought. Each has its connections and opens to new ones, sometimes to the research question. What wasn't a patch before becomes one, gets underlined in a journal, becomes a marginal notation. Others fade away. Classroom ethnographer Louis Smith returned to Cambridge for a spring leave, long into his biography of Nora Barlow, granddaughter of Charles Darwin and keeper of Darwin's papers. This trip he pondered the influence of Nora's becoming a mother and the meaning of the term *worthie*. (It meant a respected, accomplished person.) Some of his chance encounters became patches, competitors for mention in the biography. Reflecting on his search, Smith (2008) wrote "The Culture of Cambridge: Found and Constructed." He considered the patch structure of his inquiry. He said,

> The University Library grew well beyond the Manuscripts Room. The tea-room took on a life of its own. The catalogue of books and periodicals, in its old green "pasted-in" volumes and in its newer computerized form, opened the wealth of materials available to any interested scholar who has been able to obtain an admission card. The miles of stacks and the multiple other niches—reference room and rare books room—contained treasures beyond imagination.

Smith was exuberant about this ancient college scene, but he was also saying that any inquiry can be enhanced by asking the person sitting next to you what something means or reading an extra footnote. "The culture of research," Smith observed, "is both found and constructed."

CHAPTER 9

Action Research and Self-Evaluation

Finding on Your Own
How Your Place Works

A great part of your life and mine is spent informally paying attention to how things are working—around the home, around the office, and around the classroom. Or not really paying attention, just straightening things up and making it easier to do it next time, without much thinking. But sometimes we work hard at figuring out what is wrong: watching more closely, ruminating, asking for help. Action research is a lot like that. It starts with evaluation. Something is not right. It leads to studying yourself, the resources, the people you work with. It is not discovering a cure for cancer. For me, it is at the level of getting access to research sites or trying to print out mail survey addresses. But it can be a much larger evaluation of one's own organization. Often it is working with the same ideas of last week and last year, maybe trying a different way to understand the way it works or does not work. Like much qualitative research, much of it is following common sense, trying to be deliberate and disciplined about it.[1] To do it well, as described by Donald Schön (1983) in *The Reflective Practitioner*, is hard work. This chapter is about inquiry into how things work in your own bailiwick.

Action research usually starts with a practitioner realizing things could be better and setting out to look carefully in the mirror. The practitioner could be a technician, a nurse, perhaps a coach. Managers and leaders study themselves too. Often, it is one person acting alone. Often, participatory action research is carried out by one person, working with other people. It could be a team or family looking at itself. Sometimes they get the help of a more experienced person or a trainer. Many action researches, worked alone, never get known about. In many organizations, the "human resources" people encourage individual staff members to get into action research, with or without associates. Of course, it does not matter much whether or not it is called "action research."

Action research has another history, that of protesting and confronting decisions of managers or the constraints of an authoritarian culture. Such studies became well known with the anti-authoritarian work of Kurt Lewin, Ron Lippitt, and Ralph White (1939). The more recent research has been reviewed by Australians Stephen Kemmis and Robin McTaggart (2006). A fine dissertation was conducted by Markus Grutsch (2001) in collaboration with fellow doctoral student Markus Themessl-Huber at the University of Innsbruck. Grutsch started as an external evaluator of the Friends of Remedial Education, a Tyrolian social service agency. Their work together evolved into participatory evaluation (Greene, 1997), the workers becoming concerted in their press for organizational change. At the end, they were engaged in action research.

---

[1]In a paper on the history of action research, educationist Arthur Foshay (1993) described efforts before and after World War II to get teachers to study their classrooms. They were encouraged to use experimental designs and standardized tests. The few who published their action research were ridiculed by members of the American Educational Research Association, declaring the teachers naïve. The professional researchers did not recognize then—as we have in Chapter 1—that research can be based on and developed through professional knowledge, the knowledge of doing one's work. It does not have to be aimed at scientific knowledge.

9.1. PARTICIPATORY ACTION RESEARCH

If you think of research mostly as gathering information or generating knowledge, you may be deceiving yourself. Research involves information and knowledge, but most often it is coming together with others in a social milieu to better understand how something works. To emphasize the social interdependency, Kemmis and McTaggart (2006) called it "participatory action research." Action research is the study of action, often with the intent to lead to better action, but it is special in that it is carried out by the people directly responsible for the action. That could be a social worker or it could be the White House staff. It is self-study, with emphasis less on philosophizing than on performing. Asking: What am I doing? What should we be doing differently?

Box 9.1 is Kemmis and McTaggart's (2006) description of a participatory action research project in Yirrkala, Australia. Such action research is a mixture of inquiry, advocacy, and agitation. Different researchers will proportion the ingredients differently.

Self-study is to be found everywhere. Accreditation of institutions and programs sometimes includes a form of self-study. Before the accrediting agency takes up the reapplication and records available, it sometimes asks the institution staff to do a self-study. All too often, this responsibility is farmed out to a small committee or consultant with little all-staff deliberation and inquiry. These deputies too often assemble self-promoting materials and write a self-congratulatory report intended to assure good standing. But the philosophy of accreditation is that staff members will benefit by preparing a report for visiting reviewers as much as they will benefit from what the visitors have to say. When done in the spirit of community, accreditation is qualitative research and problem solving aimed toward corrective action.

Action research is self-evaluation. If initiated by someone else but carried out by the practitioners or members, it is likely to be called "participatory evaluation," still with emphasis on what can be learned and improved by their studying themselves (Patton, 1997, often included within his "utilization-based" evaluation; and Jorrín-Abellán, 2006, a dissertation study). Next we take note of forms of evaluation other than action research and participant evaluation but still important for understanding self-study.

BOX 9.1. Yirrkala Action Research

During the late 1980s and 1990s, in the far north of Australia in the community of Yirrkala, North East Arnheim Land, Northern Territory, the Yolngu indigenous people wanted to change their schools. They wanted to make their schools more appropriate for Yolngu children. Mandawuy Yunupingu, then deputy principal at the school, wrote about the problem this way:

> Yolngu children have difficulties in learning areas of Balanda [white man's] knowledge. This is not because Yolngu cannot think, it is because the curriculum in the schools is not relevant for Yolngu children, and often these curriculum documents are developed by Balanda who are ethnocentric in their values. The way that Balanda people have institutionalized their way of living is through maintaining the social reproduction process where children are sent to school and they are taught to do things in a particular way. Often the things that they learn favour [the interests of] the rich and powerful. Because when they leave school [and go to work] the control of the workforce is in the hands of the middle class and the upper class.
>
> An appropriate curriculum for Yolngu is one that is located in the Aboriginal world which can enable the children to cross over into the Balanda world. [It allows] for identification of bits of Balanda knowledge that are consistent with the Yolngu way of learning. (Yunupingu, 1991, p. 202)

The Yolngu teachers, together with other teachers and with the help of their community, began a journey of participatory action research. Working together, they changed the white man's world of schooling. Of course, sometimes there were conflicts and disagreements, but they worked through them in the Yolngu way—toward consensus. They had help but no money to conduct their research.

Their research was not research about schools and schooling *in general*; rather, their participatory action research was about how schooling was done in their schools. As Yunupingu (1991) put it:

> So here is a fundamental difference compared with traditional research about Yolngu education: We start with Yolngu knowledge and work out what comes from Yolngu minds as of central importance, not the other way 'round. (pp. 102–103)

(cont.)

BOX 9.1. *(cont.)*

Throughout the process, the teachers were guided by their own collaborative research into their problems and practices. They gathered stories from the old people. They gathered information about how the school worked and did not work for them. They made changes and watched what happened. They thought carefully about the consequences of the changes they made, and then they made still further changes on the basis of the evidence they had gathered.

Through their shared journey of participatory action research, the school and the community discovered how to limit the culturally corrosive effects of the white man's way of schooling, and they learned to respect both Yolngu ways and the white man's ways. At first, the teachers called the new form of schooling "both ways education." Later, drawing on a sacred story from their own tradition, they called it "Ganma education." Yunupingu observed:

> I am hoping the Ganma research will become critical educational research, that it will empower Yolngu, that it will emphasize emancipatory aspects, and that it will take a side—just as the Balanda research has always taken a side but never revealed this, always claiming to be neutral and objective. My aim in Ganma is to help, to change, to shift the balance of power. (1991, p. 583)

Source: Kemmis and McTaggart (2006, p. 583). Copyright 2006 by Sage Publications, Inc. Reprinted by permission.

9.2. EVALUATION

The evaluation of a national program, the National Youth Sports Program, was described in Chapter 5. Even though it only ran a year, the study was large, carried out by five external faculty researchers (Stake, DeStefano, Harnisch, Sloane, and Davis, 1997) and several graduate students. As a qualitative program evaluation, it gave readers a vicarious experience of being there, showing the program's quality in different ways and taking up several social and educational issues. The issue of conformity versus independence for camp operations, as well as for instructors and youth, was a key issue but one that led to termination of the evaluation by the Advisory Board, which rejected the methods and the intent to study the Board's functioning as part of the evaluation.

Program evaluation is methodologically different from personnel evaluation, product evaluation, and policy evaluation—but all of them are searches to recognize and report on quality of the program's working. There is a thing being evaluated, sometimes called the "evaluand." The evaluand is an evaluated thing such as a cell phone service, a summer camp coach, a drum corps performance, an admissions policy. Even in a short study, one tries to know the evaluand's activities, its physical properties, personnel, costs, and organization.

Quality is seen differently by different people, so in evaluating we need to consider various views of the evaluand. Finding different views is not a sign of invalidity of the evaluation—although evaluations can be invalid—but multiple viewpoints can be thought of as an arena, an argument, a dialectic, in which new understandings of the evaluand and its quality may be discovered.

Quality is often very difficult to discern, and sometimes more difficult to explain. We may break it into parts, to analyze the quality of the outcomes, the quality of the process, the quality of the staffing, the setting, and other provisions—yet the sum of the quality of the parts may not stand very well for that of the whole.

To make evaluation practical, many people substitute subordinate questions for the search for quality, questions such as:

Is the program in compliance with obligations?
Does the program meet the needs and expectations of clients?
Is the program productive?
What works?

All of these questions may be important, and they help move us toward an understanding of quality, but they are not the central quest of evaluation, which is, "What is the quality?"

As part of the professional practice of teachers, social workers, nurses, and accountants, evaluation is an act or a responsibility to assess the performance of people, to grade it. Even the nondirective counselor and the critical friend examine the work of "the other," informally, intuitively, seeing it as of a certain quality, and useful for taking the next steps. A little bit like God. In Genesis, it says, "And God made the beasts of the earth according to their kinds and the cattle according to their kinds, and everything that creeps upon the ground according to its kind. And God saw that it was good." It doesn't say that God had to measure anything. It doesn't say that God had to identify some criteria. It doesn't say that God had to create standards. God saw it was good. Practitioners, too, look at their own work and the work of others and see it as having reached some state of goodness. Formally or informally, they are evaluating.

Teachers examine student work and know that it is their duty to turn in grades that tell which students are doing better work and which poorer. Comparisons, rankings, or happy faces are much easier than substantive acknowledgment of quality (e.g., good organization, illustration, and sense of context). It has become convenient for educators to think of evaluation of student work as no more than testing them or ranking them one way or another—perhaps with letter grades. Most educators have come to associate the word *evaluation* with the formalities of norm referencing, even though one of the things they respect about themselves as teachers is their ability informally to recognize directly the quality of the work that students do.

Informal evaluation and formal evaluation are frequent and similar acts in contemporary life.

9.3. STUDYING YOUR OWN PLACE

It is quite appropriate for researchers to study their own places. A lot sometimes is needed to establish confidence in the findings of a self-study or the evaluation of a unit supervised by the researcher. Better design, longer study, more triangulation are part of what is needed.

The greatest concern people on the outside have about self-study is that it will be self-serving, self-protecting, promotional, advocating the home point of view. And much internal and institutional research is just that, and the institutional, corporate ethic of the modern world fails to condemn brash self-promotional research. (It is common also for a client to expect researchers to avoid raising questions that might embarrass them.)

There is a midstream choice for the researcher between (1) studying the action further and (2) getting busy at changing the action. It is tempting to move quickly into making the changes that appear needed, but it should be tempting too to dig into the matter longer to get a better understanding.

A study of one's own place is characteristic of research for the professional doctorate. With notable exceptions, the professional doctorate is not usually considered a scholarly research degree. Examples are the Doctor of Education, Doctor of Psychology, and Doctor of Engineering degrees. Most of these doctorates do require extended research, but the value is expected to be for a particular professional practice rather than for science. Thus it is appropriate for a school superintendent to study her own school district with regard to a particular issue, such as deficit spending or negotiating racial strife. These are topics suitable also for PhD research, but for the EdD, there would usually be little effort to generalize to other districts. It is also true that most quantitative studies aim at generalizable findings and fit the expectations of the PhD degree. And many qualitative doctoral studies are particularistic rather than generalizable in their findings. It should be noted that many graduate schools do not pay attention to this distinction.

> Places make us—let's not imagine that once we're here, anything else does. First genes, then places—after that it's every man for himself. . . . The fascinating thing most likely though is now the same places—a miserable school, for instance, with rotten teachers—bores one man into art and drives another into crime—the only two arenas we really have: art, making: crime, taking. . . . But doesn't that mean that people make us? Of course, but people are places. (Saroyan, 1972, frontispiece)

9.4. BIAS

Bias is ubiquitous and sometimes undesirable. Underrepresenting student achievement, seeing management as essentially conspiratorial, and failing to recognize racial discrimination are examples of undesirable researcher bias. Becoming a researcher, especially for a person doing qualitative research, is partly a matter of learning how to deal with bias. All researchers have biases, all people have biases, all reports have biases, and most researchers work hard to recognize and constrain hurtful biases. They discipline themselves, they set up traps to catch their biases; and the best researchers help their clients and readers to be alert to those biases, too.

Speaking at my retirement symposium in 1998, Michael Scriven said, "Bias, the lack of objectivity, is by definition a predisposition to error. . . . It would be hard to think of a more significant reason, a better reason, for wishing to improve our qualifications [as researchers] in the objectivity dimensions" (Scriven, 1998, p. 15). Those are words we all should study. I have not finished studying them. I hope you will take the challenge.

For there to be objectivity, for there to be a lack of objectivity, there has to be a truth. We can accept the truth of the statement that there are 10 people in the room—acknowledging that one of them might be pregnant—but we accept 10 as the objective truth. We have more difficulty with the truth of the statement that this doctoral student is ready to do dissertation research. If the committee says so, we will accept it, but the truth of the readiness has not been established. There is no evidence that will make this readiness a truth prior to the conduct of the research. We are comfortable relying on the informed but subjective judgment of the committee members.

It is about the same with surgeons being ready for an operation. We want to believe in truth that they are ready. But there is no evidence anyone can give us that they are ready. They are trained, experienced, rested, sober, and sympathetic. The surgeons themselves are confident, but even as the anesthetics are applied, they themselves do not know whether they are ready. They may be as close to ready as they know how to be. They cannot know whether they are ready. The objective truth is not available to us. Or, as I prefer to see it, because no one can know it, there is no objective truth to the readiness of the doctoral student or the surgeon.

There are many bits of knowledge important in human affairs for which there is no objective truth. And yet we study them: the safety of the security system, the danger of oversimplification with PowerPoint presentations, the imminence of Alzheimer's, the letter of recommendation written for you by your advisor. We can find good information about these things, how they work, and we can get views of experienced people and experts. But it is difficult to make objective statements about conditions now or in the future concerning the four examples mentioned here and many others.

You may prefer to believe that there is truth beyond our ability to see it. That is a common belief, and I don't urge you to change. And Scriven's advice fits that belief. We all believe that it is good to study the situation and to read the best information we can find. Michael has been a longtime reader (and sometime critic) of *Consumer Reports*. And we know that both the studying and the asking will bring us both more objective and more subjective interpretations.

Bias is also the lack of appropriate subjectivity. We would be unwise to ignore the subjective statement of the surgeon's readiness. We are unwise to disregard the hunch of the security officer. We need to include our intuitive feeling about how praiseworthy will be the letter of recommendation. We rely on experience, advice, our own biases, to weigh the subjective information available to us. We should not be too swayed by objectivity's reputation.

But the most important thing Scriven (1998) said at my retirement was that bias is a predisposition to error—an inclination to err more than it is the resulting error. In his presentation he went on to claim that there will be error in our data, some of which we can clean up and some we cannot. But the training we need to give ourselves is not so much to clean up our perceptions, our beliefs, our biases, but to minimize the effects that those biases will have on our research. How do we do this? Again, with better designs, triangulation, and skepticism.

We will try to recognize and constrain our biases but go further to check the data gathering and analyses with validation, particularly with reviews by critical friends, and by helping our readers to recognize the work that emerges still biased. One initial strategy for dealing with bias is explication, that is, making some of the important things more explicit than we have before. That means getting it down on paper or up on the screen so it can be circulated, scrutinized, and wrung out. It means taking great care to define terms and operations. It means to try out data gathering again and again in advance and to open the use of instruments and protocols to critical review. It means to be objective, allowing the least influence of personal preference. It also means allotting a large part of the budget to planning, standardization, question development, data presentation formats, and trial runs. And, for some people, it means formalizing the process of comparing measured performance with explicit standards.

I am bothered by heavy emphasis on explication and standardization. I see those as nooks and crannies where bias hides. As I said before, I want both objectivity and subjectivity to thrive. Where truth can exist, we need to measure well. Where subjective viewing can add to the depth of perception, it should. In either case—and Michael Scriven would agree—we need to help the reader see the biases we are trying to deal with.

9.5. ASSERTIONS

The conclusion of a qualitative research paper usually will feature an assertion (possibly several) about a key issue, probably closely related to the original research question. Often it is more narrow than the original question, but it could be broader. There may be mention of different perceptions or interpretations of the issue. Usually the researcher will concentrate here on the interpretation he or she finds most logical or useful or original or elegant. It cannot help but be influenced by some of the writer's bias, but it can be stated so as to invite other interpretation. Here is an assertion from the Year 1 report of our evaluation of NYSP (Stake et al., 1997):

> Operational management of the national program was effectively conducted by the director and his staff and by the chief [internal] evaluator and his colleagues. Relationships between the National Office and the [regional] evaluators on the one hand and the Advisory Committee on the other were hierarchical, [with] little healthy interactive management. The Advisory Committee showed a deep concern for the well being of the local programs and particularly for the well being of the youth but showed less concern for the well being of NCAA. They appeared not to recognize the need for patronizing those people within NCAA who have serious doubts about continuing NYSP sponsorship. Losing NCAA would be a monumental loss to these youth services. Our observations were not extensive but we concluded that there was insufficient interrelationship between NYSP and NCAA. (p. 252A)

Other assertions in the report were about quality of the local projects, student characteristics, and NYSP policy issues. Most of the assertions were relational and commendatory. My next example of a formally stated assertion is from a study of the national drum corps by Terry Solomonson (2005). He wrote:

> There appears to be a growing number of drum corps participants who return to the high school and college environments as teachers, determined to conduct their programs with the same intensity and style, without honoring or accepting the diversity of other performance programs as necessary for a successful curriculum. From a sociological standpoint, there is an apparent danger that students who are not capable of participating fully in drum corps–style curricula will be ostracized by both the student body

and the music faculty of these institutions, just as it is an apparent danger that other forms of instrumental music will be de-emphasized for the more "glorified" performance of drum corps to the point where they will no longer be provided in most schools. (p. 29)

It is sometimes feasible to insert a thoughtful rumination (a patch) from one's research log as an assertion of the difficulty one has had in gathering data on the issue. One example from a researcher's log started as follows:

> One of my main questions is about the researcher role. I am involved in a study in which my role is really embedded. I have lots of faces in this research. I am a mother of a child who attends school in the district we are studying. I used to be engaged to a man who works in the district. Now I'm not. All circumstances have had a role in my work. It would be disingenuous to claim that none of these circumstances color my vision of what is happening. But I'm not sure how to present myself. I mean, I tell all the participants in the research that I have a child in the district, and when I was engaged to the person, I told everyone that was the case. That's only respectful, I think. But when I think about what is happening and what I see, and the implications, I am torn. And I am certainly torn when I think about presenting my work. I don't want it to be discredited on the basis of my involvement, nor do I want to represent myself as a disinterested party. That would be a lie. But it would also be a lie to say that my ill-fated romance has had a negative influence on my vision, or that my positive evaluation of the education my son is receiving has had a positive influence on my vision. I like to think that I see what I see—but I know that what I see must be colored. Somehow.

Many researchers would not want to put such a personal statement in their research report, but the researcher's thought here was that the reader would be helped by considering how the multiple roles would affect what she would see and how she would report it.

One last example, this again of a small study. Rita Frerichs (2002) studied a soybean farmers' guild that contracted with individual users to deliver grain that met high specifications.

> Guild farmers are a group of larger, more progressive producers and it takes groups like this "whose fortunes are rising," to transform society (Turner and Killian, 1987, p. 247); but the Guild is attempting to work cooperatively in a world that is still hierarchically arranged (Craig, 1993). Guild

members have changed their mindset but the culture they are working in hasn't. Processors are as rationally interested in making a profit as farmers but processors have more power and backing behind them than farmers. As Enid said, "Let's face it. We can't compete with the Cargill's and the ADM's. As farmers we don't have deep pockets like they do. (p. 32)

Assertions are not summaries of the whole study but a sharp statement of an issue or condition that sums up one part of the study, perhaps summarizing what the researcher has concluded about the research question. These statements have been developed from objective and subjective data. They have had their meanings challenged through member checking, formal reviewers, and critical friends. They represent what can best be said in a qualitative voice.

CHAPTER 10

Storytelling
Illustrating How Things Work

You want to say how something works. You want to say it in words people understand, but also in words to be respected by other researchers. Researchers have the freedom to talk in many ways, including quoting other people, from sages to practitioners to children. Many people have ideas as to how the thing is working, and even the apocryphal may lead to understandings. As a researcher, you do not have the privilege to invent stories, but your perception of how something has been working can be told in story form, including the stories other people tell you. Storytelling is part of the craft of the qualitative researcher.

Some qualitative study is fundamentally the capture of a story. Not only the story of a person or group, but also the story of an organization or social movement. The recording and publication of oral history is such a venture. The story or history is seen to exist, and the researcher's job is to dig it out, interpret it, and make it available to others. Musicology, particularly ethnomusicology, sometimes uses a story form for presentation of its findings. In her dissertation on urban music, Brazilian Walênia Silva (2007) wrote:

> Dave's guitar learning at the Institute lasted about 8 months. After that, he practiced on his own and played professionally in a local group. Four

years later, he was invited to teach a course at the Institute. He went on to more courses and private students. He considered teaching as a possibility to make a living. He was motivated to teach for two reasons: money and Frank Hamilton. He described Hamilton's course:

> They played "On Top of Old Smokey" and "Freight Train, Freight Train," two of the oldest, most dusty songs, but he got people playing. And things were happening—harmony. Later he and I had a cup of tea and I said, "I wish I could teach a class like that." He said, "You can!" "But I don't know enough about music." "What's that got to do with it?" he replied. "You begin, you ask questions and then you work to answer them. If it's too hard, do something simpler. Isn't that right?" (p. 122)

The story was about learning to play folk music at the Institute of Urban Music in Chicago—group immersion, just playing, no scores. The story is alive with experience as told by Silva, who learned to play new instruments there and adapted the techniques for school music in Brazil. That's how the thing worked in Chicago. That's how things might work in Brazil.

10.1. VIGNETTES

Sometimes our stories will be brief, a snippet in time, contributing little to experiential knowledge but bringing to life an issue central to the research or one that illustrates the complexity. Some of us call these snippets "vignettes." Box 10.1 is a vignette that poses one of the deepest of

---

BOX 10.1. Twins

"You taught Sammy how a camera works, but you didn't teach Sally."

"But Mrs. Johnson, Sally needed to do her math."

"It isn't fair."

"I love them both. I wouldn't be unfair."

"Sally hates math. Can't you make school as good for her as for Sammy?"

"They are different kids."

"You should be equal for both."

ethical issues, the choice between meeting educational requirements and making opportunity for children equitable.

The issue being illustrated with a vignette is not always obvious from it. Most of us are reluctant to explain our jokes to people, but we have an obligation to explain our vignettes. Here the teacher considered it appropriate to reward the child who had completed his math assignment, reinforcing his high performance. But the mother thought less of production than of making school attractive to a daughter with perhaps less mathematical ability. Both seem attractive aims, but competing.

As illustrated by anthropologist Frederick Erickson (1963), qualitative research assertions are sometimes illuminated with vignettes. A vignette is a verbal illustration of response to a research question, not necessarily generalizable, sometimes poignant. As in Box 10.1, it can be a wisp of dialogue. Sometimes it grows beyond anecdote to something of a short story, such as the bubble gum experiment, but usually it is short. It may be but the trace of action, such as the shadow of lipstick on a photo on the piano. Momentarily it is "figure," but shades into the "ground" of a larger issue.

Consider the issue of transition services for youth with disabilities wanting to gain employment. School-to-work transition services are limited. Not all the community's eligible youth can be admitted into a small preparatory program. Some selection is necessary. Advocacy groups have acknowledged five priorities, such as admitting first (1) those youth most recently out of high school, (2) those youth with the more severe disabilities, (3) those youth predicted to show greatest gains in employability from the program, (4) those youth most eager to participate, or (5) those youth with homes most distant from social services. It was an issue in a qualitative research project (see Box 10.2). The vignette and the research project do not need to resolve such issues. It is good research if it clarifies the phenomena, the activities, the setting, and the issues. A qualitative vignette does not need to indicate how common the happening is, although the researcher may take steps to find its typicality. The assertion in this instance might have read something like:

> Concern for program productivity sometimes runs counter to equity. Being equitable may be costly. A project honoring equity may appear less success-

BOX 10.2. Transition Services

There was one opening in the program. Aimie applied. After leaving school she had lived with her parents, without a job but helping at home. Earlier she showed interest in the Transition Project, but it was 25 miles away. In the past, rural girls had somewhat less often than rural boys completed training and taken a job offered. Aimie's parents worried about her wages cutting their welfare payments. Aimie had been on the "eligible" list for 6 months. Frank was new to the community, wanted work badly, was unable to find a job for himself, appeared to take the situation seriously. Mentioning a first-come, first-served priority, Aimie was invited to enroll. The program would be evaluated partly on the basis of the number of trainees it placed in employment.

ful at placing trainees into employment and keeping them employed. With equity, the funding goes less far because of expenditures for dropouts and low performers. In the program studied, the rhetoric was egalitarian, but recruitment efforts and encouragement were unequally distributed among those who showed low and high likelihood of placement.

Let's look at another vignette, anonymized (Box 10.3).

BOX 10.3. Relief from Pain

I was not part of the ward staff the day before and was not familiar with the patient, but I explained to the mother that it is possible to do the procedure without sedation and that I was sorry that it had not worked, but with sedation today, Lennie should be settled enough to have it done successfully. Having looked at Lennie's drug chart and noticing the absence of analgesia, I indicated to Lennie's mother that she could ask the doctors to prescribe pain relief for after the procedure, as very often patients can be sore at the site of needle insertion and can suffer headaches. . . . To this she replied that she had requested pain relief the day before. However, the doctor did not chart it, no nurse requested it be charted, and therefore Lennie received no analgesia following the failed procedure.

10.2. ELEMENTS OF STORY

The traditional form of story is, first, an introduction of characters and context, then the revelation of problems that stir apprehension, increasingly complexifying, and ending in good or bad resolution of the problems. It is a chronology, as if going from "Once upon a time" to "And they lived happily ever after," with an occasional flashback. That format, of course, is quite different from the traditional research format that goes from statement of the problem through review of literature, data collection, analysis, and interpretation. The story form is an alternative presentation, preferred in some research places. But even in the most traditional places, a story usually can be used within some sections of a report.

There are those who advocate just letting the story tell itself (Coles, 1989; Denny, 1978). That means the particular situation calls out what will be described in detail and valued. And that implies that the researcher should arrive ready to listen, with little priority of information needed, accepting of the frame of reference and interest in detail of the people there. It sometimes works. As indicated throughout this book, however, the researcher usually has a research question, a plan of data gathering, and patches of testimony already gathered, and he or she takes a risk in letting the storyteller decide what story to tell. Usually, the researcher will pose some questions, possibly refer to other stories, and interrupt adroitly to move the story in ways that fit the research design. The researcher's strategy can range from open ears to a highly structured asking for stories.

The style of the qualitative researcher is empathic, respectful of the reality portrayed by the storyteller. Still, usually, more will be asked for than was volunteered, and less will be reported than was told. It is most often the researcher who will decide what leads to understanding of the phenomena of interest. The report will be the researcher's dressing of the teller's story. Any criteria of representation are the responsibility of the researcher.

Qualitative research is holistic research, detailed, rounded, contextual. We would like to tell the whole story. But we cannot tell what exceeds page limits and audience patience. (If you are a tree in the forest, you know that what isn't read wasn't written.) And there is always more story than anyone knows.

Next, an example of a qualitative research story. The professional people running the International Step by Step Association program wanted to know the accomplishment and diversity of its developments in preschool education across Eastern Europe and Central Asia. They commissioned a multiple case study, cases in 29 participating nations.[1] For each case they selected two to four of their own experienced teacher trainers as the researchers and let the program director from each country choose the research question or theme.

"Inclusion" was the theme of a case study in Ukraine—inclusion particularly of children with disabilities. The research team, Svitlana Efimova and Natalia Sofiy, chose to tell the Step by Step story in their country by selecting Liubchyk, a child with a disability mainstreamed into a regular first grade taught by a Step by Step teacher. Liubchyk was diagnosed as having autism. He attended Maliuk School near his apartment in L'viv. With Liubchyk as the hub of the study, they moved out the spokes to study teacher training, parent involvement, and the media, plus relations with local and state education authorities, including the Ministry of Education and Science. The complexity of Ukraine's changes from having an institutional special education system toward an inclusion practice was illustrated by numerous observations and interviews. (The graphic design of the case study is shown in Figure 10.1.) We saw one observation of Liubchyk in Box 3.2. Box 10.4 is another observation report of his classroom.

The professional knowledge gained in Ukraine and in the other 28 countries included generalizations about Step by Step preschool teaching in countries across a large sector of the world, but of course not generalization to all preschool education in the world. The particularities referred to classrooms such as Liubchyk's and to the Ukrainian Ministry of Education. Many readers of the assertions in the Ukrainian report would generalize them to other teacher training agencies and ministries. And they would presume the applicability of many of the findings of the cross-case report, such as the value of teacher training that occurred in actual kindergartens with Step by Step trainees role-playing as teachers of the pupils belonging to that room. Here we see generalizations and particularizations living side by side, as they will in the minds of practitioners, policy specialists, and beginning researchers, mixing research knowledge with professional knowledge.

(text resumes on p. 179)

---

[1]This case study is presented in full and analyzed in my book *Multiple Case Study Analysis* (Stake, 2006).

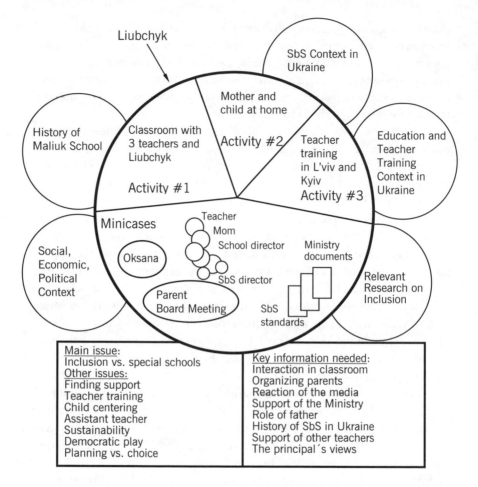

FIGURE 10.1. Graphic design of Ukraine Step by Step (SbS) case study.

BOX 10.4. Liubchyk's Classroom

The next assignment for each child is to color a printed scene from the fairy-tale, Thumberlina, and place them in the order the scenes appear in the story. The children work in groups. Seven-year-old Liubchyk chooses a picture among those offered by Halyna, the assistant teacher, but he refuses to join a group. He is not pressed to do so. "What is this bird?" she asks. Liubchyk spreads his arms and says, "A swallow." "Very good," says Halyna and pats him on the shoulder. The children work their scenes. When the coloring is completed, the children gather and the scenes are laid out in order. "Liubchyk, come here, we are missing your picture," says his friend Anychka. Liubchyk gives her his neatly colored swallow but continues to stay close to Halyna.

A year earlier, although he wanted to come to school, Liubchyk would talk neither to teachers nor children. Now he was talking to the two teachers and his social worker and interacting on occasion with two girls who regularly befriended him. His teacher, Oksana, had originally opposed passing Liubchyk from kindergarten to first grade, but upon getting better acquainted with him and his mother, and getting further into Step by Step teacher methods, she accepted him and became an advocate for mainstreaming. Resisting to a small degree the advice of a consultant, Oksana gave him considerable freedom to join and withdraw as he chose.

The researchers studied Step by Step teacher training in L'viv and also in Kyiv. They observed trainees working in a mainstream class and they observed trainee groups studying attitudes toward inclusion policy. For example, with the Four Corners exercise, one sign was placed in each corner of the room. The signs identified four alternative organizing principles:

1. Children with special needs must attend the same classes with other children if they are capable of mastering the same material.
2. Children with special needs must attend special schools that provide for their specific educational and medical needs.
3. All children regardless of their abilities must attend regular classes.
4. The parents of children with special needs must decide which school each child will attend.

(cont.)

BOX 10.4. *(cont.)*

Olga, the trainer, asked the participants to read the signs, then to go to the sign that best expresses their own opinion. The participants moved about, reading the statements. Sign 1 drew the largest group, and Sign 2 the smallest. The discussions are based mostly on personal experience. "My neighbors have a child like that. . . . " "I have a child in my mainstream class but the parents do not pay attention to the child." Olga rings a small bell and . . . invites spokespersons to take the floor.

The history of organizing an inclusion advocacy group was explored in a long interview with Volodymyr Kryzhanivskiy, the director of a parent-based health-improvement center. He was an engineer, father of a boy with cerebral palsy, and sought equal education for him. Put off and put off until, on the advice of an official, he and fellow advocates formed a nongovernmental organization (NGO), Shans. Ultimately, inspired by Hospital 18 in Moscow, they built a center for assistance and education, not only for children with disability but for parents, other caregivers, and advocates.

Efimova and Sofiy wrote in detail about the tradition and legislation of child care in Ukraine. Following Communist ideology, all children were to be educated, but those with disability were hidden from the public, in boarding schools or possibly at home, treated according to diagnosis but denied the experience of growing up with ordinary children and teachers. Slowly, today that inequity is being recognized. That professional specialization created a large cadre of diagnosticians and caregivers who opposed mainstreaming because it left too dispersed the care they were trained to give. Had this study been continued, it probably would have inquired into the care of children at those special schools.

Still working the story centering on Liubchyk, the authors described the work of the Ukrainian Step by Step Foundation, detailing its programs, capacity, and partnering. Gaining Ministry authorization for teacher training and funding for assistant teachers were prime aims. The director said:

> It all started in 1996 during the International Outreach Meeting of Step by Step in Prague, where the initiative on inclusion of children was announced. . . . In the summer of 1997 we . . . invited officers from the Ministry of Education and Science. . . . It was difficult for them to understand and accept the idea of inclusion. They saw risks to the existing system of specialized institutions.

(cont.)

BOX 10.4. *(cont.)*

In 2003–2004 Ukrainian Step by Step evaluated their inclusion initiative and found that the children with disability were successfully engaged in the state curriculum and that the rest of the children also benefited from the experience.

Step by Step gained the support of the Institutional Building Partnership Programme of the European Union and got its license from the Ministry to train teachers—but funding for assistant teachers continued to be obtained only locally. In ending the report, the authors included these words in their assertion on the mainstreaming of Liubchyk:

> For Liubchyk's mother the opportunity to bring her son to Maliuk School was a great relief. It strengthened her belief that everything with Liubchyk could be worked out. Clearly, it was an alternative to the decision of Pedagogical–Medical–Psychological Consultations to send him to a specialized institution. Liubchyk is a very interesting child. He has unique skills. Hearing her words brings out a picture of a gifted child, a very special child indeed. But this is the essence of inclusive education. Each is skilled. Each is special. Education is available for everyone, including those with gifts of every kind!

Source: Efimova and Sofiy (2004). Copyright 2004 by the Open Society Institute. Reprinted by permission.

10.3. STORY VERSUS A COLLAGE OF PATCHES

How do you conceptualize your own study? A few qualitative studies can sometimes be thought of as unfolding stories. The phenomena or cases being studied continue to develop and engage new contexts. The researcher links their development to the passage of time, seeing them as contemporary history. Still other qualitative studies are more the story of the researchers, a person or team investigating phenomena, episodes, or cases. Each of those is an autobiographical account of that particular inquiry. But studies of these two kinds are unusual. It is unusual for the research to be told strictly as a story, even though it has a strong chronological structure and detailed accounts of problems and resolution. Usually qualitative research will be more effectively perceived as episodes, patches sewn together by ideas, not a story of researchers in data sites. The projects will be seen as a succession of topics, as descriptions and interpretation of events, acknowledging the researcher as data gatherer and interpreter but not a main character in the play.

Managing your research project will be facilitated by keeping in mind a selection of patches: key observations, photographs, vignettes, and interviews, the ones most likely to appear in detail in the final report. That comes naturally, but you can work to do it more productively, more elegantly. (Patches are imagined in Figure 8.2.) At the same time, partly from the circle graphic plan (Figure 10.1), you will be thinking more and more about what may be your topics in the final report. For Ukraine, the patches and topics are shown in Figure 10.2. In qualitative research comes the opportunity to perceive the study as a collage of patches,

20 Patches

Liubchyk comes to school	Liubchyk helping the teacher
Ms. Oksana	His mother's advocacy
Step by Step standards	Questions from reporters
Stories in the newspapers	The Four Corners exercise
Alexander and Ann	Ministry of Education
Ailsa Cregan, a mentor	Volodymyr interview
Board meeting	The special "internat"
Soviet policies	Ogneviuk interview
Zasenko interview	Sofiy interview
Thumberlina	The swallow

16 Topics

Liubchyk	Liubchyk's teacher
Teacher training in L'viv	Press conference in L'viv
Teacher training in Kyiv	Teacher training in Ukraine
Liubchyk's mother	Shans, a parent NGO
National context	Legislation
Treatment of children with disabilities	Ukrainian Step by Step Foundation
Partners	Views of education policy
Views of teacher training	Views of inclusion

FIGURE 10.2. Patches and topics for the Ukraine Step by Step study.

structured by experience and contexts. But there is safety and stability in seeing the research as a story or progression from research question to assertions. Perhaps you can have binocular vision.

10.4. MULTIPLE CASE RESEARCH

The Step by Step research just described was a multiple case study project. Embedded in the plan were 29 country case studies. Many of those country cases had one or more minicases embedded within them.[2] In the Ukraine study, for example, Liubchyk was the main case, and his teacher was studied as a minicase, as was the Shans, a parent organization supporting children with disability. Here is a bit of dialogue at a Shans board meeting (from the final report):

> MS. MARINA (a young mother): We have to give more attention to developing the habits of self-help. We should enable a child to learn household things—how to cut, how to use the phone, things like that.
>
> MR. LJUDA: We parents strongly want to "hypercare." I understand it. I struggle with it. I go to a neighbor's house and painfully sit for 30 minutes, leaving my child alone at home.
>
> MS. MARINA: I had no alternative with my child on crutches. I said, "If he wants to survive, he will survive." I need to earn my living. I was leaving him to care for my daughter, 18-month-old Dimka.

An important message for the Shans parents to the professional staff was to make the teaching of "independence from disability" as important as the teaching of reading. That issue was not brought up in the other Step by Step case studies, partly because inclusion of preschool children with disability was less a priority in most of the country stories.

Parent involvement was a priority in all the countries. It was an issue to be drawn together from all the cases. It was identified as an issue before the multiple case study started. I have used the term *quin-*

---

[2] The International Step by Step program could have been considered a "macrocase." From the quintains across the 29 cases, the researchers made macrointerpretations. But in the single Ukraine case, it was Liubchyk who was "embraced."

tain to identify an issue that runs across the cases (Stake, 2006). Parent involvement in teaching was a quintain for the Step by Step study. In the analysis of such a study, an interesting struggle arises between the case-specific issues, such as teaching independence, and issues that are the quintains. The case researchers do not want to give up the assertions they carefully developed, whether or not they are found elsewhere. The cross-case researchers want to keep attention on the assertions common to most or all of the cases. It is an intriguing competition, with the professional view more apparent in the individual cases and the scientific view more apparent across the cases.

Quantitative research methods, however they borrow from mathematics, have grown out of the search for the grand theories of science. To make generalizations that hold over diverse situations, most social science-oriented researchers make observations in multiple and diverse situations. They try to eliminate information that is merely situational, letting the contextual effects "balance each other out." (Contextual effects are such influences as poverty, religion, promotional policies, and the like—unless they are the effects being studied.) Quantitative methods deliberately nullify contexts in order to find the most general and pervasive explanatory relationships. "Generalization" is what we call repeatedly found relationships between variables, such as dependence and disability; between parental age and teaching independence; between all the factors studied in social science and professional work.

Most formal social research is characterized by this search for grand explanation. Controlled measurement and statistical analysis, that is, quantification, have been used to permit simultaneous study of large numbers of dissimilar cases, in order to put the researcher in a position to make formal generalizations about social phenomena. To study Alzheimer's disease or to study police leadership, most researchers seek as large a sample as they can get.

For policy and theory, we look to macroanalysis. For understanding how things work in general, we need the methods that lead to generalization. Usually that is quantitative study. But we also need to understand how individual things work. The needed truths are sometimes in the things in front of us. For that, we need the disciplined study of the particular.

CHAPTER 11

Writing the Final Report

An Iterative Convergence

People have different styles of writing, and yours is probably good for you. Content is more important than style in the final report.[1] The task of organizing the content is important in preparation for the final writing. At least in your mind, you have, in some ways, been organizing the content as you gathered data, made preliminary interpretations, considered its value as evidence, and stored it away. Perhaps you have boxes and have allocated pages. Some of your patches are ready for the first draft of the final report. Your intuition is at work. This is enough for some people to sit down at the keyboard and begin the final writing.

But other people need additional organizational structure, some sort of formal scheme for pulling together those data now partially analyzed and interpreted. You may be one of the people whose assertions and collection of patches need a final organizing.

We can use an iterative process drawing from the intellectual power of the research question and the experiential power of the fieldwork. We can use the two powers for reconnoitering and setting aside the weaker ideas. We would examine the evidence for each orientation, thinking how each leads to better understanding and assertions.

---

[1] Good thoughts about publishing a report are to be found in David Silverman's *Doing Qualitative Research* (2000) and in Donileen Loseke and Spencer Cahill's "Publishing Qualitative Manuscripts" (2004).

For the final report, you have many ideas to put together. Synthesis should not be primarily a matter of presenting them all, in order of importance or in clusters, but reaching some new, composite, integrated understandings by considering all the ideas together. We do something like that in ordinary thinking, intuitively contemplating, for example, the whole of a conference, an emergency room, or a vacation. But intuition can be supported by a formal iterative strategy. And that is what the following iterative procedure is supposed to do.

11.1. THE ITERATIVE SYNTHESIS

To iterate we need to make outlines successively approximating the final outline for writing the report. Each step requires thought. I like to think of it as digging down to the meanings of the study, but Iván Jorrín-Abellán told me it was better to represent the iteration as in Figure 11.1. Note that some outlines are closer to the research question(s) and some closer to the fieldwork patches. Think of us having moved through the research project following two grand plans. We have followed two intellectual pathways. You have been sensitive to them along the way, although you may not be able to identify them at this moment. One is the plan to answer the research question. That is, to reach a greater

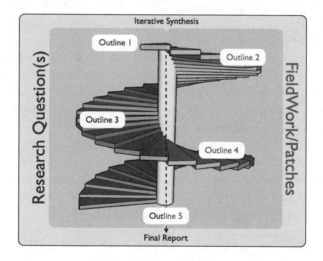

FIGURE 11.1. Iterative synthesis of an outline for the report.

understanding of the topics, relationships, problem, and content closely related to the research question. The other plan is to work from the collection of patches, from the descriptions of happenings and the perspectives encountered in fieldwork. We often think of these two plans as one plan, but they lead to at least somewhat different conclusions.

Each plan is a search for patterns, for consistencies, for common meanings. Some patterns are patterns of inconsistency. The qualitative research question, as you work with it, becomes more complex, not less, more situated and seemingly dependent on its context. Moved by the question and issue development, it may increasingly appear that, for example, (1) how the teachers teach will be influenced by the availability of chairs or (2) mainstreaming requires a backing away from performance standards. These may be patterns that become more apparent by relying on the research question to push the data gathering and interpretation (Bourdieu, 1992).

Other patterns can become apparent by rereading and rearranging the patches, the key incidents, the themes. For example, (3) chairs were essential to one teacher's behavior control, and (4) the parents of children in Liubchyk's class repeatedly offered support for the teacher. Of these four patterns, which should get top priority in the report? The iterative procedure will help determine the priority of topics and issues by their value to the research question and their standing among other patches.

To begin the iteration, you concentrate on the strongest topics and issues and weed out the weakest for understanding the research question. Then you do a similar sorting according to the ways the patches hang together, almost without considering the research question or original topic development, leaving out those that yield the poorest evidence of how the thing worked. Then back again to selecting those best supporting the research question, leaving more out, and again, for maybe two more iterations.[2]

The synthesis is something of a dialectic, a thrust and counterthrust, an intellectual resolve of competing forces. As indicated in Sec-

---

[2]Perhaps I should have proposed early in the book that you prepare for this iterative dialectic, but I felt that there were many things with which to become familiar first. The power of the patches may not be felt until you have some. The thrust of the research question may not be appreciated until you get further acquainted with it during data gathering.

tion 11.4, we start the research with a lot of wandering thoughts, but then we settle on a main research question, or two or three. We may refocus that question later, maybe more than once. The research questions may be complex, needing more than a paragraph to state. Such questions are advance organizers, serving as a structure for our data gathering and interpretation. In the Ukraine Step by Step study, the question led us to the boy Liubchyk. How could we come to understand his learning and his autism as a first grader? But the research was also about the child-centered alternative pedagogy developed by Step by Step in Ukraine. The research questions were complex but helped keep the observing, interviewing, and document reviewing moving toward thematic targets. That was the research question plan, the upper pathway of Figure 11.2.

The competing plan was to come to know the places and events of the sites and data sources. The research proposal identified a number of sites, data sources, contexts, and episodes to come to know in depth. The proposal acknowledged that they are complex, manifest with human purpose, and strained by social issues. The qualitative methods used invited rich description, recognition of multiple realities, and labored interpretation. The events encountered were not contained by the research question; they stretched beyond. They invited our consideration of alternative research questions.

In Ukraine, the researchers in the field found that the teacher training was brief and filled with advocacy for inclusion and mainstreaming. The mission of the program included public relations and petitions to the Ministry of Education. The response of Liubchyk's classmates to his self-indulgence was caregiving more than distraction and confrontation. There were many stories to tell. There were many patches to assemble. Should some patches be prominent in the report even if they were not good evidence for the research question? This iterative convergence did

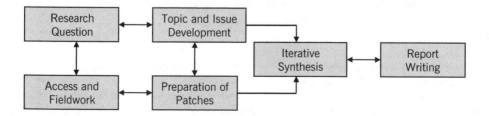

FIGURE 11.2. Dialectic flowchart from question to report.

not answer that question but gave us ground for making the final collection of patches and interpretations.

To do such a dialectic, you need to outline your final report once for each iteration—perhaps using the boxes (Figure 4.3) or the assembly plan (Figure 8.4), reshaping it each time, a little or a lot. The first outline should be based on your research question(s). And then do the second outline by thinking how the report could represent and make understandable your collection of patches. You have two outlines, created separately, the top two shown in Figure 11.1.

You think again of the research question and how the first outline might be improved by adding things from the second outline, merging and omitting some. The modification becomes the third outline. Next you take the second outline, still emphasizing the patches, but add and merge some things from the first outline, omitting a little of lesser importance among the patches. You make the fourth outline (for the final report) more sensitive to the research question than the second was. Then you compare the third and the fourth outlines carefully and create a fifth as the best this study can put forward. The final outline is not determined by the research question or the patches, but by your judgment of what you have most to say to the reader.

Such an iteration could have been done much earlier, in the initial planning, and during writing up of field notes, between chapters or at planned intervals. The summary message of your report will not be equally based on the research question and the fieldwork data; there will be a leaning toward how you see the phenomena you studied.

Speaking of such an approach as naturalistic, Robert Emerson (2004) described how one researcher (the esteemed Howard Becker, 1961) worked gradually, iteratively, to develop an incident during hospital rounds into an assertion of how medical students viewed patients. It was a matter of reinterpreting while data gathering. Emerson ended saying, "Naturalism requires ethnographers to develop theoretical propositions *during and after* immersion in the field." I would consider Emerson's description and his quote both as patches.

To use such a naturalistic dialectic, like Becker, you avoid the idea that there is one right assertion (or one right report), some optimal integration of the research question and the fieldwork. And become comfortable with the idea that the final report can be driven most either by the fieldwork or the research question. One of the leanings might not be acceptable to you or to your boss or to your doctoral committee, but either can be a respectable research synthesis.

11.2. THE UKRAINE REPORT

Let us illustrate the iteration using the Ukraine study. Its research question might have been stated, "How has the International Step by Step program developed in Ukraine in the years 1995–2005?" A second research question might have been, "How did the Ukraine Step by Step program make it possible for Liubchyk, a boy with autism, to be a first grader?" The circle plan for the Ukraine study was shown in Figure 10.1. The boxes (issues and topics) and patches for Efimova and Sofiy's Ukraine report were presented in Figure 10.2. We now use the iteration procedure to practice making an outline for writing their final report. (We already know the Ukraine researchers, early in their research, decided on the outline and page allocation shown in Figure 11.3.)

We would study the Ukraine research questions carefully again, noting main concepts and, with a mental concept map, examining the related topics. We might put each topic on a card to move around on the table. After realigning these topics, possibly discussing them with colleagues, we might say that the main content (as oriented to the research question) for the final report should be (1) child-centered teacher training, (2) inclusion, (3) children with disabilities, (4) parent support, (5) equal opportunity, and (6) legislative policy. That is Outline 1.

Next we would study the patches and recall the experiences of the fieldwork, making a new set of cards. Putting them in order of the prominence we would like to see them have as representations of the phenomena studied, paying almost no attention to the research question, we might select this distribution of content for the final report: (1) teacher training, (2) advocacy for change, (3) inclusion, (4) the nature of autism, (5) social learning in school. That is Outline 2.

Returning to a consideration of how the research question might best structure the report but wanting the field experience to be prominent, we would use the second outline to modify the first. The new priorities (Outline 3) might be: (1) child-centered teacher training, (2) Liubchyk, (3) inclusion policy, (4) advocacy for change, (5) autism, (6) parent support. The next outline would use Outline 1 to modify Outline 2, still emphasizing patches but heeding the research question more; thus Outline 4: (1) Liubchyk, (2) inclusion policy, (3) disability of children, (4) teacher training, (5) social learning in school, (6) advocacy by parents. Finally, 3 and 4 would be merged into Outline 5, perhaps moving teacher training a notch higher.

Topic Sections	Pages	Pages of context	Questionnaire info	Inclusion	Teacher training	Child-centered educ.	Democratic play	Program sustainability	Choice vs. standard	Insertions of Patches from Zone 3	Zone 3: Patches	
											Other topics	Quotes, impressions
Liubchyk	5			X			X			D,C,3	1. teacher selection	A. Black today, green tomorrow
Oksana	3	1		X	X	X			X	F,1	2. child protection	B. Director not bureaucrat
Teacher training, Aviv	3	1	X	X	X					4	3. child view of disability	C. Liubchyk's view of time and management
Press conference, L'viv	2			X			X				4. teacher view of disability	
Teacher training, Kiev	2				X						5. nature of disability	D. body contact
Teacher training, Ukraine	2	2		X	X						6. role of church	E. teacher staffing vs. potholes
Liubchyk	3		X	X						3	7. teacher unions	F. Oksana's activity centers
His parents	2		X	X							8. European Union TACIS	G. parents voted support
Parent Organizations	2	2		X							9. Chernobyl effects	H. psychological assessment
LEA, Aviv	2	1								B,9	10. special education alternatives	I. aggression, affection
Ministry	2	2		X		X	X				11. preparing parents	
SbS Ukraine	2	2		X		X	X		X	2,8		
Interpretation: Alternate education policy	4					X				10		
Interpretation: Teacher training	4		X		X							
Interpretation: Inclusion	4			X						E,5		
Liubchyk	2			X						A		
Total	44	11										

FIGURE 11.3. Assembly plan for the Ukraine final report.

These priorities do not indicate the order or size of the topic in the report. These terms might or might not be headings of the sections of the report. All that can be done with the page allocation form (Figure 8.4). In Figure 11.3 are the names of topics and the allocation of pages decided on by the researchers, Svitlana Efimova and Natalia Sofiy. In the "Topic Sections" column for Ukraine are roughly the topics just identified. After being told by Step by Step officials that the report should be 45 pages long, the two researchers decided they wanted to give 10 pages to the description of Liubchyk. But also they wanted, as you can see, to start with Liubchyk, to have some middle pages on him, and to end with him. Most of the patches they anticipated would have an experiential flavor, as in what you read about Liubchyk in Chapter 10. They wanted almost a quarter of the report to be about the boy, even though they had considerable obligation to write about Step by Step across the whole country. They wanted the reader to experience him as a person and to be conscious of him while reading about teacher training, parent involvement, and the issues of inclusion and national policy.

The Ukrainian physical and political contexts were important. Liubchyk's community was not far from the nuclear disaster at Chernobyl. Many children had suffered disabilities. A quarter of the pages, 11 out of 44, were apportioned to context, spread out over seven sections of the report. You are following this in Figure 11.3, aren't you?

Even more explicit than with many programs, the Step by Step organization called for political advocacy. The teacher trainers were to press the Ministries of Education to be more supportive of preschool in general and of "alternative" pedagogies, particularly child-centered teaching. Their professional view was partly a political and media view. The Ukraine researchers chose to hold a press conference on the issue of school inclusion of children with disability and then, in planning the case study, to observe and record it for the report.[3]

At the time that Efimova and Sofiy first conjectured their assembly plan, they had no patches. But, 2 months later, they had 11 brief topics and 9 quotations. These patches gradually were assigned to the topics identified in the left-hand column. Liubchyk's clothing suggestion to the

---

[3] The Step by Step people caused news stories to be written about school inclusion of children with disability. Their internal researchers, in a sense, were in a position of creating and reporting the news. They acted professionally. It might have been unethical had they hid this promotional commitment from their readers.

assistant teacher—"Black today, green tomorrow"—was assigned, as shown, to the final two pages of their report.

The assembly plan can give the researcher an early overview of the developing study and prospective report. In the Ukraine plan, the scientific view was not highly visible partly because the main research question was surrounded by many competing questions. Rather, a professional view was strongly supported, with alternative themes and observed episodes getting many of the pages.

To structure the report with greater priority on the research question, Efimova and Sofiy could have used their report's first section to identify the Ukrainian Step by Step program and the issue of inclusion in primary education. Liubchyk probably would have been described in one section rather than three. The research question was given high priority in the next to last three sections, devoted to their interpretations, closing with attention to inclusion. The authors wrote the report, discussing it themselves and with me, then circulated drafts for reaction. Some reviewers pressed to have more said about other sites of Step by Step activity in the country, but the pages were strictly limited, and the patches describing episodes in and around Liubchyk's school held their place.

11.3. DUALITIES AND THE DIALECTIC

You may sense that this dialectic and iterative approach has been important to me in writing this book. I have proposed a number of dualities in previous chapters.[4] Hopefully some of them will come back to you as you employ the converging dialectic:

- Qualitative and quantitative research.
- Macrointerpretation and microinterpretation.
- The general and the particular.
- Scientific knowledge and professional knowledge.
- Collective and individual knowledge.
- Aggregative and interpretive data.
- Measurement and experiential understanding.

---

[4]Dualities can be simplistic, stereotyping complex matters, but they can also be a starting point for looking at differences.

- Single and multiple realities.
- Analysis and synthesis.

Both sides of each duality can be found in our dialectics. The research question pathway and Outline 1 will probably get more macro-interpretation, possibly some emphasis on the general and scientific knowledge, and will attend more to collective and aggregative data. The fieldwork patches will probably get more microinterpretation, clearly an emphasis on the particular and on individual and interpretive data, possibly some attention to professional knowledge. (It will seldom help to sort the patches and topics into these categories, but it can help to think, "Are my Outlines 1 and 2 drawing from these dualities as much as I would like them to?")

Let me say again that using these graphic forms can be a long "work in progress." You sketch them early and revise them as the fieldwork continues. Yes, there is likely to be a particular time when you sit at the keyboard saying, "Now I have to write it up." But, hopefully, you have a lot of patches already drafted. Of course, there still are lots of decisions to be made about format, illustrations, style, bibliography, and so forth, but you want to make it most clear to the reader what you were looking for, what you did, what you found, and what you make of it. In other words, how the thing worked.

Organization theorist John van Maanan (1988) spoke of seven choices of presentation: realistic, impressionistic, confessional, critical, formal, literary, and jointly told—lots of choices. But the choices are limited by funding agencies, prospective readers, rhetorical convention, prospects of publication, hospitality received, the researcher's colleagues and career pattern, and more. Some criteria for how to write a report are set by notions of what will best answer the research question. Some commitments are made when the study is designed, and some are made while the last spelling check is spinning along.

11.4. PARTICULAR AND GENERAL ASSERTIONS

One of the dualities, the particular and the general, should help us think through how we want to state our assertions. Do we want an assertion to refer to the specific phenomena studied or to be asserted more generally? As we work through our observations and interpretations, and as we near time to collect all the pieces we have written, what have we to say? We provide the reader with vicarious experience. We select the best of our interpretations of the phenomena. We have new notions as to how things work. And we punctuate these with a few assertions. We sometimes extend our assertions toward generalization and at other times concentrate those assertions on the particulars we have studied. Of course it depends on the evidence we have gathered but, usually, some of both.

As you may remember, in this book's early chapters, I contrasted the general and particularistic. I offered them as trade-offs, my favorite dualism. I posed them as opposites to increase the tension, to magnify the differences, because I thought it would help you understand things. But now I want you to face the reality that both the particular and the general coexist in all the things we do, in the thoughts we have, in the reports that we write. For example, I think of each of you as individual readers, and, at the same time, I think of all the readers who might read these words. At this moment you may be thinking of me as a lone writer lost in a forest of murky ideas, but simultaneously as one of many writers having too few of your needs in mind. Here together are the particular and the general—as in Figure 11.4. Any one report that you might write may favor specification or generalization but will contain both. I believe your assertions need a dollop of each.

In a page or so, I quote poet William Blake raging against generalization, but he also wrote (in "Auguries of Innocence" edited by Walter Feldman):

To see a world in a grain of sand
And heaven in a wild flower,
Hold infinity in the palm of your hand
And eternity in an hour. (1982a/1997)

The micro and the macro coexist. The scientific and the professional coexist. The particular and the general are different but are to be found together.

Whatever a report will say, it will say different things to different readers, some seeing more of the particular description and other more of the possibility of generalization. Another line from Blake (in "The Everlasting Gospel") went:

Particularistic Assertions	General Assertions
1. This office and the agency's central office have arrived at different perceptions of the reorganization plan.	1. The perception of reorganization varies from center to periphery in social service agencies.
2. The summer retreat was used more to solicit loyalty and compliance than to provide continuing professional education.	2. Training meetings are being used more to solicit loyalty and compliance than to provide continuing professional education.
3. Last year, this school of music increased its offerings to assist students to prepare to give instrumental band instruction.	3. The job market for musicians who can give instrumental band lessons is narrowing the curriculum in college schools of music.
4. Women staff members here made twice as many protests about the new rules on seniority.	4. Women are more willing than men to take risks that might jeopardize their job security.

FIGURE 11.4. Examples of particularistic and general assertions.

Both read the Bible day and night.
But thou read black where I read white. (1982a/1982b)

Among your readers' expectations is that the report could be a guide to setting policy for situations such as those studied. Also possibly expected is that the report could provide people with vicarious experiences so that they can deal better with similar situations they will encounter. Those two expectations may sound the same, but they are not. They correspond to our interest in the general and the particular, to the macrocosms and the microcosms, to the quantitative and the qualitative. Since ancient Greece, scholars have debated the relative worth of general knowledge and particularistic knowledge.

Socrates and Plato pursued the "grand meanings" of worldly affairs, generalizations that might serve to improve the laws, communications, and customs of people collectively. Most often, the physical sciences and social sciences have followed a similar aim, elevating grand theory and holding individualistic personal, professional, and public experience as a subordinate level of knowing.

Aristotle acknowledged that grand, collective, impersonal knowledge can help to deal with worldly affairs but, taking issue with Socrates, said that people cannot avoid relying on the knowledge of their own past experience. Prudent handling of the large and the small in life requires attention to the particular values of each situation. And the meaning of each situation is related to situations even earlier. Many generalizations are rooted in personal experience, not so much drawn from what people have said. (Deborah Trumbull and I [Stake and Trumbull, 1982] called them "naturalistic generalizations.") The more important of these experiential roots need to be remembered in detail and in context. Just as much as abstract generalization, experiential knowing is essential to the epistemology of individual people and agencies. The study of human activity often loses too much value for practitioners when the reporting primarily tells what is common among the several and universal across the many and too little of the individual and personal.

Aristotle did not call it "prudent knowledge," "purposive knowledge," or "experiential knowing"—he called it *phronesis*. Philosopher of science Bent Flyvbjerg used Aristotle's term too. In criticizing Socratic social science and researchers' hankering for grand laws to guide human affairs, Flyvbjerg (2001) said:

> *Phronesis* goes beyond both analytical, scientific knowledge (*episteme*) and technical knowledge or know-how (*techne*) and involves judgments and decisions made in the manner of a virtuoso social and political actor. I will argue that phronesis is commonly involved in social practice, and that therefore, attempts to reduce social science and theory to *episteme* or *techne*, or to comprehend them in those terms is misguided. (p. 2)

In his book *Making Social Science Matter* (2001), Flyvbjerg claimed that social science has been insufficiently helpful to human problem solving. Its intent to generalize has contributed too little to fixing what is not working.

The weakness of traditional science for studying an individual person, group, episode, or policy was put forth long ago, and again by Barry Mac-Donald and Rob Walker (1977) and by Robert Yin (1981). Knowledge of the particular flows from an inquiry tradition described by Georg Hendrick von Wright (1971) as the search for understanding. We talked about it in Chapters 1 and 3. You probably figure it's old hat by now. Researchers, lay persons and philosophers, and professionals often need to know the particularity of a case, its situationality, and its social context.

I am fond of particularization, but another quote from William Blake goes too far. In "Annotations to Sir Joshua Reynolds's 'Disclosures,'" he said:

> To generalize is to be an idiot. To particularize is the lone distinction
> of merit. General knowledges are those that idiots possess. (1808/1982,
> p. 641)

Why would he say that? I don't understand. Every thinking moment has
its generalizations. No two experiences are entirely different. As soon
as we have two, we start to expect something in a third. We generalize.
Although we sometimes overgeneralize, we sometimes undergeneralize.
Keeping the balance is important. Particularization and generalization,
in balance. Balance doesn't tell you what to do next. Do all summer
camps offer kids experiences they don't get at home? Summer camps are
sometimes held in a home. And sometimes we want to understand how
an atypical summer camp works. For writing good reports, we need a
discipline of the particular as much as of the general.

Flyvberg's disappointment with social science may be warranted—
but public expectation of science seems wired in. On into the future
will be the expectation that research is best at providing formal generalizations for guiding policy and collective practice. And also the
expectation that analysis and problem solving can be jump-started by
the structural thinking[5] of clinical psychology, medicine, education,
and other professional practices. In the beginning, social science can
help draw the design by providing descriptors and reconceptualizing
common research questions. These advance-organizing expectations
have merit, but an epistemic approach sometimes undercuts the valuable understanding that the phenomena are unique and situated. Even
though approximating a truth, cognitive generalizations are often too
abstract and too decontextualized to guide practice. Still, epistemic
thinking is as natural as it is artificial, so we strive to keep it connected
to practice.

It is expected that epistemic generalizations are based on enduring
relationships and can be used to predict the effects of change in practice.
Scientific generalizations continue to be respected in research communities and administrative circles. But they are problematic in that they
lead to expectation that they optimally facilitate professional practice.
Most practitioners agree that targets and limits of practice for a profession may be established through epistemic generalization. Measure-

---

[5] Structural thinking is what we find in statements of rules, likelihood, functional
relationships, and categorical comparisons.

ments icon Lee Cronbach (1974, p. 14) said, "Generalizations decay." And sound choices of professional action will continue to rely on custom and advocacy.

Still, formal generalizations make an important contribution to debate and deliberation of social policy. When treated as hypotheses and working positions,[6] generalizations provide valuable counterpositions to experience and convention. Both are grist for deliberation and debate (House and Howe, 1999). *Phronesis*, *episteme*, and *techne*, each has its contribution to make.

11.5. GENERALIZATION FROM PARTICULAR SITUATIONS

Flyvbjerg (2004) wrote that one of the most serious misunderstandings of social science was the belief that case study is not useful in making generalizations about how the world works. We looked at his reasoning early in Chapter 1. We regularly work with generalizations, formal and informal, such as, "Children with autism don't like to be touched" or "People with Alzheimer's remember long-ago experiences better than recent." And then we encounter exceptions. So we modify our generalizations, making them more conditional, or stochastic, or less predictive, or we make a new generalization, or refrain from generalizing about it for a while.

A small amount of qualitative research can falsify a generalization. It is rare that a small amount of qualitative research can bolster a generalization. But that happens, too, notably in professional practice. A promotional ad for a political or sales campaign stirs a protest, and the organizer says, "I'll never do that again." But he or she will do something similar. The extent of the generality of our generalizations is regularly unclear. Even in the best of sciences, we are unsure about to what populations the findings apply. The research designer recognizes the need to include certain variability in the observations and contexts, but many variations are not included. This is true also in qualitative research. We pay attention to the diversity we have to work with. We describe that

---

[6]Note the reversal of this definition of qualitative study from what used to be reluctantly allowed: . . . but [qualitative research] may be useful in the preliminary stages of an investigation since it provides hypotheses which may be tested. . . . " (Abercrombie, Hill, and Turner, 1984, p. 46).

diversity for readers, but we also speak specifically of the likelihood that the findings would be different for other situations.

Even as we particularize, such as writing about one clinic or one firehouse, we make petite generalizations. We make assertions about it and expect they will hold at least for a little while into the future. We expect that small changes in staffing, in rules, or in financing will not turn things around. We expect that the clinic or firehouse on the other side of the city has similar complexities and similar engagement with its environment. It may not, and we have guesses as to which are the more vulnerable petite generalizations. And we talk to our readers about the limits of generalization. But we and they do expect to learn about other clinics and firehouses from studying one or a few (Ercikan, 2008, p. 207). All experience is similar in that regard. The first experience of diaper changing or kissing or graying of hair influences what we will expect in the future. We generalize. We transfer. We extrapolate. It is difficult to specify the limits or risks of the generalization, but we often generalize from particular situations.

11.6. THE PROFESSIONAL VIEW

Your final report may benefit from a professional perspective more than you have considered. As indicated in Section 1.2, professional knowledge is enriched by the separate knowledge of the professional's own field. Social work has a lore based partly on familiarity with families in distress, a lore that is different from that of pastoral counseling, which also has deep knowledge of people in distress. Social workers, community workers, psychiatrists, and priests work together, but their worldviews and technical practice are based largely on their work experience—though also partly on their professional community: its separate history of financial support, moral and sacred beliefs, and engagement in legal responsibility, for example. And subdivisions within their work—such as, for the social worker, with foster care and care for immigrants—create their own special clinical knowledges, knowledge from service in special workplaces. The professional draws upon personal experience and on the social sciences but has a professional view enriched and entrusted through the ethics and reputations of the discipline.

A professional view comes primarily from the experience of service to others, working with colleagues and teams and allied services, each having special training, routines, and sensitivities. What especially characterizes this view is the fact that how things work varies with the situation. There are the legendary professions—medicine, law, ministry, and education—with experience and understanding of the human situation, collectively and case by case. Their members decide—from observation and inquiry, from training and experience, with ethical standards—how to work within the strictures and theories they face. Similarly exercising choice in human care are the practitioners of old and new professions, the trainer, the nurse, the counselor, the city planner, the physical therapist, the psychometrist. Into what knowledge reservoirs do they reach when faced with a new problem?

Professional practice relies heavily on qualitative inquiry. However refined the methods used, it is expected that the choices of action will not be mechanically determined but must be reached through interpretation. Those interpretations will depend on the experience of the researcher, the experience of those being studied, and the experience of those to whom information will need to be conveyed. The professional knowledge of our reports relies heavily on personal experience within an organizational setting.

Some professionals remain hungry for further experience. Some do not. Agency officials and supporters want to know how things are working in various settings for which they have responsibility. They may have little confidence that your research can give them vicarious experience in as sophisticated a way as they would have by seeing it themselves. They are experienced in the disciplined study of the particular. You are aspiring to that too. And you are learning, partly from this book, how to write your final reports with a qualitative research discipline that most of them do not have.

CHAPTER 12

Advocacy and Ethics
Making Things Work Better

There is wide agreement that research should make things work better. There is less agreement that researchers should use their research to advocate for particular solutions. Some choose research questions and interpret their research so as to maximize helping things work better. We need critical studies, but advocacy spotlights some flaws and hides others. That can be a problem. Some say that the world will not be made better until we understand it better. I am dismayed when I feel that researchers are jumping too quickly from investigating into ameliorating.

12.1. ALL RESEARCH IS ADVOCATIVE

Most researchers see themselves as searching objectively for explanation and understanding. They shudder if someone says they are biased or too subjective. Many of their own mentors once said that "research should be value-free." But almost no one now believes the social researcher can operate without exercising personal values. Yet, they sometimes speak angrily of research that deliberately takes sides, promoting or opposing some cause. And still, it is clear that researchers, like other people, have strong feelings about social matters and show advocacy in their reports. Box 12.1 lists advocacies of qualitative researchers.

BOX 12.1. Six Advocacies Common in Qualitative Studies

1. We care about the groups we work with. Often we hope to see their work advanced. Some researchers are studying a part of their own organization. Barry MacDonald once said, "One should not study a program if one does not support its goals." Seldom do we have a large conflict of interest in our research, but often we have a *confluence* of interest, a sharing of interest. We hope to find the group succeeding. We are disposed to see evidence of success.

2. We care about the methods we use. We want to see others care about them. We want to encourage them to use the methods too. We sometimes promote qualitative study as a professional service to help people. We favor methods that dig into the depth of issues, and we encourage others to probe in similar ways. Our methods are an advocacy we flaunt.

3. We advocate rationality. We are comfortable with personalistic knowing and intuition, but we support rationality strongly. We would like the people we study and study for, and our colleagues and administrators on campus, to explicate and be logical and even-handed. We sometimes pause in our data gathering and reporting to point out ways that the people could have behaved more rationally.

4. We care to be heard. We are troubled if our studies are not used. We feel qualitative study is more useful if the participants take some ownership of the research. Some of us are advocates of self-study and action research. Even a quantitative study can profitably use input from constituents, including suggestions for design and interpretation.

5. We are distressed by underprivilege. We see gaps among the privileged—the patrons and managers and staff—and underprivileged participants and communities. We often devote some of the study to the issues of privilege, coming up with research questions that illuminate or possibly might alleviate underprivilege. We like distribution of our findings to reach people distant from research.

6. We are advocates of a democratic society. We see democracies depending on the exchange of good information, some of which our studies can provide. But also, we see democracies needing the exercise of public expression, dialogue, and collective action. Most case study researchers try to create reports that provide grounds for and stimulate action.

We do advocate, yet we are troubled. We are troubled by the possibility that our advocacies will cause us to search more vigorously for aspiration-focused evidence than for other evidence. We cling to some advocacies more than to neutrality, believing these well-considered biases to be compatible with the interests of the profession, our clients, and society.

Each of us is more than a researcher. We are complex human beings. Some of the things we do are part of our work and some are outside our work. Each of us has political, spiritual, aesthetic, and other advocacies. Some of the panorama of advocacy cannot help but become part of the final report, even if we individually try to separate our research assertions from the rest of our life. Perceptions and values from any part of our lives may influence the interpretations we make in writing a final report.

12.2. A VOICE FOR THE UNDERREPRESENTED

Many of us qualitative researchers aspire to work with people whose voice has little carry. For the poor, for minorities, for those with disabilities, for the disenfranchised. Our studies perhaps may illuminate the plight and virtue of the disenfranchised. As advance organizers, we express need for empathy, for assistance, for advocacy—even sometimes ignoring conventional research ethics. As a program evaluator, I remember *under*stating the shortcomings of a teachers group, thinking otherwise the budget knives might cut deep, possibly forcing its termination. And you know those stories too. Advocacy abounds. Even in our most ethical research, there is advocacy, with some of it intending to assist "marginalized" people. In studying them, many of us become their agents.

But I am not confident we serve the people we research well. How accurately do we read their need, their aspiration, their constraint? We are confident, sometimes overly confident, that the more we know about them, the better we tell their story. What is the evidence that the impoverished are empowered when we portray their impoverishment? What is the evidence that the rebellious find empathy when we illuminate their cause? I would say the evidence is weak. During the Iraq War, I read in a newspaper that graffiti on a Baghdad wall voiced the question, "Is help helping?"

Much research is sponsored by those who believe that with factual knowledge comes better policy. But we know that much social and educational policy is formed for narrow political reasons, self-perpetuating, not always to make a more democratic world. The facts are used selectively, and sometimes to deepen the plight of the under-class. With skepticism we should continue to question our rationale for studying the disenfranchised. And one of the questions has to do with the intrusiveness of the personalistic methods of qualitative research.

Yes, I question the grounds for intruding into the lives of those we would help. We want to lessen their hurt. But we serve ourselves too by taking up their cause. We serve our pride, our vanity. In our circles we are admired for our words of care, for the stories we tell.

To get to better description, we press closer to those we study. The story comes slowly. We entice and cajole and purchase. We choose the facts and quotations and mood to report. Is the expression coming from our keyboard their expression? Is it an extraction, a wrenching away, something of their private selves?

As often said in this book, qualitative research methods emphasize the importance of multiple perspectives, recognizing that there are other ways of seeing things, other ways of explaining things, and alternative ways of changing things. We need the same multiplicity of views and values when we reflect upon our own work. The first argument is that we are allies of those with little voice. The counterargument is that we do more harm than good.

The good we expect is that, working collaboratively, as Linda Tuhiwai Smith (2005) and Antjie Krog (2009) would have us do, we will enjoin educators, parents, community members, and public policy setters to reach out with respect and caring. And, in some measure, we do that. But we do harm too. We sometimes tell their story badly. We sometimes expose their condition, and contrary to our intent, we get some people to dismiss them as beyond help. We may undercut their aspirations by clarifying the enormity of the obstacles they face. We may cause them to try less. There is another. One possible harm is next on my list: violating their privacy.

12.3. PERSONAL ETHICS

The following excerpt is from a collection of case studies about adolescents in trouble. In her report, the researcher, Linda Mabry (1991), quoted a girl she called Nicole as saying:

I started getting in trouble probably the summer after seventh grade. I hung out with people that were in high school. I *looked* older, but I wasn't being responsible like an older person. I start thinking about the past like, "God, that was stupid!" Your parents say, "When you're older, you're going to thank me for this." But (back) *then*, you don't care.

Second quarter of my freshman year, last year, I moved in with my aunt upstate. Then we got in a fight over my grades. So, fourth quarter, I went and lived with my dad. While I was there, my stepmom and the two kids packed up and moved. My father and I were left together about a month, and he tried something on me. I was standing up, and he had his arms around me and was rubbing me up and down. I called a friend to pick me up. I got my checks where I'd been working, called my mom, and bought a bus ticket back home. My mom told me to call the cops, and I did but they said they couldn't do anything because he didn't get in my clothes. . . .

I've smoked pot maybe ten times. I've done speed once. I've never done cocaine or shot up or anything like that. I haven't smoked pot in probably six months. I don't need that stuff to have a good time. Some of those kids are screwing their lives up. (p. 17)

The case study of Nicole was part of a collection published by Phi Delta Kappa to portray young people failing. I agree that professional and lay people need to know about such troubled students. I did not consider it at the time, but I now think that her privacy may have been compromised. Is it ethical for a researcher to enter into an anonymized, consenting, collaborating individual's privacy? I don't know. Is it still invading an individual's privacy if the individual's identity is effectively concealed? Aren't we giving voice to youth who need to be heard? I just don't know.

I found those three paragraphs the most intimate and self-incriminating words of a 24-page chapter. They nicely represent the deep intimacy of some case studies. The researcher's care and caring were there for all to read. But just by the fact that we have Nicole's words here for all to read, how can we say that this was not a breach of her privacy?

Would we agree that life stories like this one can be of value to many readers? Yes. So we have a dilemma. At some point, getting closer is intrusive. At some point, learning the next fact about an individual will be a violation of his or her privacy. And can't the same be said about the privacy of a family, of a community, and of a people?

Some kind of "zone of privacy" exists, though not in the same way for different cases, nor for the same case in different circumstances, nor for different researchers, nor for different audiences. Privacy is relative, situational. We cannot expect hard and fast zone boundaries. They can change in the space of an hour. The shift and transparency of the boundaries does not make them less real. It is difficult for a researcher to find the zone of privacy into which he or she should not step. (What about Question 3 that ends Section 5.4?)

Each person can be expected to have somewhat unique zones of privacy. Zones for many people may be similar, but I think it necessary that we presume each person is different and changing. When a person feels threatened, the zone will be larger. When a person is sitting among strangers on an overseas flight, the zone may be smaller. We are sometimes willing to confide in a stranger something we are not willing to confide to a family member.

A researcher I know was studying immigrant families. One father was cold and unsympathetic toward his unmarried sister, who had become pregnant. His wife admitted being sympathetic toward her sister-in-law—but could not say so to her husband. She volunteered all this and explained the sequence of events that led to the illegitimate pregnancy and how the extended family members and the community at large reacted to the family's plight. The wife also asked that this not be mentioned to her husband. If her husband began talking about his sibling, then the researcher was asked to behave as if she was hearing it for the first time. "He will get really mad at me for telling you," she said. "It matters a lot to him how you think about our family, and this news is not good news at all." The researcher did not particularly want to hear about it and did not include it in her report.

You may be thinking that it is not a violation of privacy if Nicole or the immigrant wife volunteers the information, that where the informant sets the privacy boundary should be the law. But sometimes the researcher may need to set an earlier boundary. None of us can be counted on to know, each time, what information we should keep to ourselves.

In a long-ago evaluation of computer-based learning, Barry MacDonald was interviewing a headmaster, who said: "I wish they would send all these black boys back to the Caribbean." Barry said that he could not include such a quote in his report. The man told him something like, "Well, you should. That is honestly the way I feel." A year or so later, unrelated to the opinion he had expressed, the man was seeking another position. It might have been useful for the potential employers to know what Barry knew. But was it his responsibility to tell them? He thought not. I think not. Shouldn't the principle be that we researchers need to honor privacy even when our informants fail to? Unlike with doctors and attorneys in similar situations, our silence is not protected by law. But shouldn't our ethical principles call us to remain silent? (For much more on research ethics, see Ryen, 2004, and Mertens and Ginsberg, 2008.)

12.4. PROTECTION OF HUMAN SUBJECTS

In the history of social and medical science, there have been a few research studies that seriously injured people, and many more in which their welfare was not sufficiently protected. Nations and research associations have taken steps to prevent hurtful and intrusive research. Human-subjects review boards have been established. On American university campuses, we call them institutional review boards, IRBs. They have authority, they have a mission, they do some good; certainly they are no substitute for personal care by researchers.

Rules of ethics give inadequate protection against violation of ethics. Just to continue being the nice people we are gives inadequate protection. Review boards are too far removed from the research to give adequate protection. The people being researched cannot be counted on to protect themselves. It is the researchers themselves who provide the bulwark of protection. Through empathy, intuition, intelligence, and experience, we ourselves have to see the dangers emerging.

In social research the dangers are almost never physical. They are mental. They are the dangers of exposure, humiliation, embarrassment, loss of respect and self-respect, loss of standing at work or in the group. The probability of hurt may seem so low that researchers contend that the potential good of the research to society outweighs those small dangers. Some have spoken even of a "right to know." It is important to find out how things work. But is there any scientific, political, or public right to know that justifies a single case of intrusion into personal privacy or threatens personal standing? What do you think?

Human-subjects review boards operate differently from country to country, even from campus to campus. Each country and institution and research team should follow strong review procedures for conducting human research. Uniform procedures have been officially adopted in the United States, but so far, in my view, they have been inappropriate for qualitative research and ineffective in protecting human subjects. Norman Denzin (2002) has evaluated the situation well in his chapter on "Performance Ethics" in *Pedagogy, Politics, and Ethics*, noting both orientation of IRBs to biomedical research and their overreliance on "informed consent." By requiring full planning in advance, the American IRBs interfere with the evolving nature of action research, case study, and participatory evaluation. Ethical conduct of interpersonal research depends not so much on letters of informed consent but on deliberated and collaborative caution by the researcher, invoking a demand for help from critical friends (McIntosh and Morse, 2008). These review board problems can be fixed, but until they are, we need to obey the law while we heed our own higher standards.

To return to the matter of privacy, the researcher should not rely on the informant alone to identify the intrusion but should work at anticipating it along the way. Avoiding intrusion should not be thought of as satisfied by maintaining confidentiality. Anonymity is weak protection. The main way to respect a person's privacy is not to come to know the private matters. The researcher should not solicit private information that is not closely related to the research question. For impersonal matters, the inquiry can evolve spontaneously. But for highly personal matters, solicitation should be announced well in advance.

In the United States, during the Clinton presidency, there emerged a problem of how to deal with gay men and women in the military. The rule adopted was, "Don't ask. Don't tell." Perhaps in our world we should do better than that. For us, perhaps it should be "Don't ask. Don't tell. Don't listen." When someone starts to reveal a private matter, should we say, "Ah, that is a topic we need to put off for now"? Should we say, "I'm sorry. We really have time for just one other critical question"? Or should we knock a cup of coffee into our lap? Almost anything to avoid the zone of privacy.

Box 12.2 presents some possible rules to diminish intrusion. It is incumbent on the researcher to anticipate it. Some of the rules have more of a privacy aspect than others. It may help us keep in mind a zone of privacy like the one mentioned earlier.

The problem of intrusion is important yet little addressed as part of research design, triangulation, and training. Conventional readings

BOX 12.2. Rules to Diminish Intrusion

1. Regardless of where data are to be gathered, "personalistic research" will enter the "spaces" of personal experience. The researcher needs to get close enough to comprehend that experience and stay far enough away to avoid intrusion into the truly felt private.
2. Access to those "spaces" is not through a one-time "letter of consent" but a continuing negotiation of roles and permissions to inquire about matters, personal and otherwise.
3. Personal access sometimes needs to be given formally by persons in authority but always by a continuing showing of willingness by each participant. The researcher needs to develop acuity to read those signs.
4. Termination options should be clear. Exiting should not be taken for granted.
5. There is a special problem when the data provider is under obligation or pressure to participate but is not fully willing. The researcher needs to weigh the costs of going ahead, with or without discussion with this data provider.
6. In dealing with highly personal matters, children and others in dependency should have an advocate present during initial negotiation of access and possibly during data gathering.
7. Early on, the research proposal (or an abbreviated but not deceptive version) should be made available. Previous pertinent reports by the researcher should also be accessible. The main research question(s) and the specific topics to be raised with the person usually should be indicated.
8. When disclosure of the aim or a topic would possibly alter the behavior of the person and hurt the research, that information should be given to his or her advocate in advance and to the person, as part of member checking, after data collection and well before writing a final draft.
9. By pledge and in showing respect, the researcher should give the person reason to believe he or she can be trusted to avoid putting people at risk or burdening them.
10. Even beyond the extent asked, the researcher should indicate, in writing, who will have access to raw data and how the interpreted findings probably will be used.
11. If the researcher is funded or is serving an advocacy effort, the sponsors and other associates should be identified.

(cont.)

BOX 12.2. *(cont.)*

12. Usually, beyond token gifts, the researcher has little, other than gratitude, with which to pay a data provider. He or she should not offer benefits that research often fails to give. He or she should not pose as therapist or problem solver.
13. The role of the researcher as (a) stranger, (b) visitor, (c) initiate, or (d) insider-expert or other (see Agar, 1980) should be thought out and indicated.
14. The researcher and the person being studied can together become collaborators, but the benefits and responsibilities should be carefully and repeatedly explored, sometimes with legal counsel.
15. The researcher should have a plan for data gathering, intuitive or formal, which again undergoes scrutiny for protecting human subjects prior to each data gathering.
16. Advance into new and unexpected personal topics should carry a warning.
17. When a person begins to volunteer personal and private information not directly pertinent to the study, the researcher should interrupt the revelation and divert the inquiry—and sometimes even when the information is pertinent.

of methods often offer us simplistic and nonexperiential warnings. Each of us has to plan for each situation. If we leave it to intuition, however good that usually is, we may hurt people. And on the triangulation side, the quality of our data often depends on making and keeping good personal relationships. We need to remember that, at the end of the study, whatever understandings we have gained may not be worth the trouble we have caused.

12.5. PEOPLE EXPOSED

The reality of personal fieldwork is very complex (Lee, 2000). A cultural divide between researcher and researched appears even when gathering face-to-face data in a neighboring community or in an unfamiliar organization or just in a new house down the street, but we are less worried about how to behave among those strangers. With an intention to learn across cultures about patterns of belief and behavior, in matters personal and private, the estrangement can be considerable.

When is permission enough? I will tell you about a privacy problem that I faced in 2003 and again in 2006 when I was writing that book on multiple case study analysis (Stake, 2006). The book included three Step by Step case studies, one of them in Slovakia. As you read earlier, in some 30 countries, Step by Step was primarily a teacher-training program for child-centered kindergartens. But in Slovakia, the primary attention was on inclusion—particularly on the education of Roma children, who were not being admitted to first grade because their cultural backgrounds were not scholastic and they spoke Romani rather than Slovak, the language of the schools. The program developed a home-based teaching program, getting mothers and grandmothers (who themselves knew little Slovak, or how to hold a pencil and identify a triangle) to teach their children. The women were coming, bringing their preschool children 1 full day a week, all of them getting instruction. And in the remaining days of the week, they would instruct the children at home.

The Slovakia Step by Step Foundation leaders located their research study at one of their projects in a Roma settlement adjacent to the village of Jarovnice—where the efforts had been quite impressive. For more than a year, mothers and children had been coming to the Community Center and the Pastoral Center for instruction. They were supported by a tiny staff of Step by Step teachers. One of the vignettes from their case report is in Box 12.3.

With some help from me, the researchers wrote up a 40-page case report of this Jarovnice project. It was really good. I got their permission to publish it.

But, as I have said, permission is not necessarily enough. I published the report. Still, should I even have been a party to describing the history of the meanness to and the poverty of these Roma families? I cannot automatically agree with those who say, "Their story needs to be told." They greatly needed help. The stories might help. But also, the stories expose them, put them on exhibit. And I do so again in these pages.

In Slovakia we were dealing with violation of personal privacy and the privacy of a people. It was their settlement being exposed. Should our research ethics allow us to expose their conditions? As in almost all ethical problems, there is a choice between two ethics. Which is more important here, portraying the conditions or avoiding the hurt of exposure?

BOX 12.3. Case Report Vignette

At the Community Center, 14 Roma children ages 6 and 7 sit around Iveta Fabulová, their teacher, in the corner of the room, to hear a story about Marika. Nine Roma moms have joined them.

Iveta tells them all a story about Marika, a Roma blacksmith's wife. "She had too many children, and they didn't have enough to eat. One day her husband put shoes on a horse for a farmer, and the farmer paid him with a sack of flour. Marika took the flour, added water and baking soda, and made dough. She slapped the dough into a flat, round shape. She baked it over the fire. The delicious smell of the bread went out to the whole settlement. It smelled so good that everyone came to Marika's house. She fed everyone. Because her name was Marika, they called the bread '*marikle*.' Ever since that time, long ago, Roma people have been baking *marikle* to remember the generosity of Marika."

The children and their moms listen to Iveta quietly. "What do you think about this story?" Her question is addressed to a mom sitting next to her. "She was a good person." "Yes," replies Iveta, "she was generous. She shared bread with other poor people."

"Children, what was the shape of the bread? Was it like this one?" Iveta takes a round loaf from a bag. "Look, its shape is a circle. Try to draw a circle in the air. And repeat after me, 'Circle.'" The children draw circles in the air and shout, "Circle!" in chorus.

"In Presov, people buy garlic bread shaped like this." Iveta points to a yellow triangle on the blackboard. "I want you to draw this triangle and repeat after me, 'Triangle.' And soon we are going to make bread in these two shapes."

Iveta invites them to choose their activity center. The children quickly move to the centers where material has been prepared (clay, paper, pencils, pens). Some choose clay, others paper and pencil, to make these shapes. Olga, a Roma woman, the teacher assistant, helps divide the clay. The mothers move their chairs to join each group. Iveta asks them to help the children name each shape. Later, Iveta says, "Do you know the names of the shapes you made? What is this, Dusan?" Dusan has drawn circles and triangles of different colors and sizes. He answers without hesitation. Many children need the teacher's help to pronounce the Slovak word for "triangle."

But there is a more personal exposure for which I have been responsible. One of the photographs taken by the team was of a mother and father at home helping the children to draw. I was fascinated by their faces. I wanted to use it as a cover photo on my book.

The Step by Step program was already using the photo as one of many in their promotions. The foundation director readily gave me permission. I said, "Do we have the permission of the family?" I was told that they are very happy to have us helping them, happy to have us show them doing their lessons, that they are proud to be doing what they are doing. I passed that word along to my publisher, but I still did not feel comfortable. And it was not just because I had no signatures on an agreement.

I asked a researcher with experience with the Roma in Romania. She said, "Privacy never comes up as an issue." "But do some of them sometimes feel that we are exposing them?" "No one speaks of it." I got the same answer from a retired anthropologist. He said, "We honor the local customs. We didn't talk about what they didn't choose to talk about. We followed their lead." Are we being helpful or intruding? I don't know. Sometimes trying to help things work better makes them not work so well. But there is no alternative to trying until there is reason to believe it is hurting more than helping.

12.6. ESSENTIALS OF QUALITATIVE RESEARCH

The report of home schooling in Slovakia[1] can be used to look back at what this book tells about qualitative research, previewed in Box 1.2. It will help us think about the typical as well as the diversities of ways to do such studies. And it will remind us of the methodological choices available, including the fact that many qualitative studies will have some quantitative thinking and data.

The report of illiterate mothers preparing their children for school had "story quality." It spoke of the experience of the women who planned and carried out the plan. Stories present sequences of problems. In this Roma community, they looked at one main problem: the social discrimination. The Roma were almost without a social support system.

---

[1]The full report of the Slovakia case study authored by Eva Koncoková and Jana Handzelová can be read in Stake (2006).

Research seemed needed to make real the destitution and the stamina, not in the language of economics but in the language of experience.

The report was interpretive, highly interpretive. It described the people, the spaces, and the activity, but it spoke of these things as they were interpreted by Roma persons, by non-Roma community members, and by the people who funded Step by Step and came to observe the social changes. These interpretations revealed multiple realities across the groups and among individuals within the groups.

The researchers identified many contexts that gave meaning to what was happening in the situation. The political and educational contexts included a long-standing lack of social and governmental support for the Roma, but later with Ministry of Education and European Union rhetoric changing toward support and the protection of diversity. The efforts of the Step by Step teacher trainers were a big part of the contextual picture.

Vignettes and photographs and quotes helped to make the study personal and the report empathic. For most readers, the community was unique, almost hypothetical, and the teaching unreal—because it departed from much of their own experience of teaching and learning— yet the mothers and teachers and children were real. The study helped make them real.

Not much was apparent of the Slovak researchers' efforts to triangulate their data and interpretations. There was little effort to relate the study to other research literature on the Roma, on post-Soviet education, on ethnic hostilities in the Balkans, on literacy, on school admissions, and many adjacent topics.

Among the choices the researchers made was to work toward practical understanding more than toward theory development. They chose not to establish the typicality of the settlement situation. They chose to support their own views of education of Roma children rather than let the descriptions stand for themselves. Efimova and Sofiy chose to recognize the multiple realities present. They worked with particular knowledge but frequently spoke of it as generalizable. And they had no inclination to keep program improvement separate from the effort to understand the situation better. Like the program itself, the research was not flawless but still produced a successful research study.

These were not experienced researchers. They were early childhood educators. They followed their instincts, their common sense, but they also worked to discipline their study. They repeated their observations, deliberately sought multiple interpretations, and pondered at length the words and ideas to include in the report. They conveyed the experience of Roma mothers in an almost hopeless situation working to help their children. Can these teacher educators be a challenge to the rest of us trying to figure out how things work?

12.7. LOOKING FORWARD

Here at the end of the ride, you have a lot to look back on. But as you know, you can look back further than Chapter 1. You have been doing qualitative research since your own kindergarten, and before. Of course, your research is better now than it was in kindergarten. It is more disciplined and will become increasingly so as you extend your experience.

Since kindergarten, you have experienced all the stuff around you, like bicycles and curried chicken, and a first date and being a stranger in a strange land, and you have figured and refigured what it means, and then you have realized it meant something else to your sisters and something else to your attorney. And there it is, multiple realities, not even the same between your sisters.

Of course, not everyone gets excited about multiple realities. And one of the important things about qualitative research is that there are so many different things to get excited about, and lots of people have a different twist on what they mean.

Looking forward, perhaps you are thinking, I don't really want to see things differently, I just want to turn the corner or to pass my quals or get a better job. How am I more ready for the interviews? They will be expecting me to have some right answers. And I have doubts that I've found enough right answers since kindergarten and particularly in this book.

So when they interview you for that dream job, the one that pays all expenses to professional meetings, you figure that you need right answers. And the right answers are some version or other of "it depends." It all depends on the situation. And you will tell them that the researchers you have read and admired have looked closely at situations, and you know that what works in one situation does not necessarily work in another, that the complexities are great, and that the Powers That Be end up setting policy based on the pressures they are under and the experiences they have had. Not just the impulses, although impulses are right some of the time. To figure what will work next takes a lot of pondering, some new data, and a lot of relating to the best cautions and assertions that practitioners and researchers have passed on to you.

Qualitative research depends on planning, but one thing you have to plan especially well is to be open to new ways of interpreting things. Being able to sketch it out. Being able to talk it through. Bringing in new interpretations that tie in with economic, political, and communication developments may be the best right answer.

The words of this book have tried to add up to a right answer to the question, What works? One answer is that different things work in different places. You know how to look closely in a particular place, better now, I hope, than when you started Chapter 1. Answers can be figured out, not often to solve a problem completely, not ones we can always fit within a budget. But we can figure out how not to keep making the same mistakes, because figuring out how it works includes figuring out how it doesn't work in the trouble we are in right now.

The problems of cultures (as in Box 12.4) and the problems of policy are not solved by research. They are tackled and sometimes ameliorated by people who draw on professional knowledge and research knowledge and talk about it with other people and work something out. It is not like building a bridge. It is not like testing a new pharmaceutical. It is thinking many times about what works in some situations and trying something better for this situation.

BOX 12.4. Ana and Issam

The kindergarten is one of three classrooms at the training center. Eighteen children are working and playing around the room.

Marja, a short woman in her 40s, is a kindergarten teacher with child care experience. Working with her today is Luci, a young trainee from outside the country. Both Marja and Luci are well aware of an ethnic split among the children, but Luci has little experience with diversity in the classroom.

Ana seizes Issam's black brush and starts to paint with it. Issam cries. Luci shouts, "Ana, give the brush back to Issam." Ana looks at Luci, then at Issam. She takes the cup of black paint and pours it on Issam's hand. "He's black!" she says.

It has been important to learn that how the thing works in several small situations does not aggregate to solving a big-thing problem. Answers to macro problems call mostly for study of macro situations. Answers to micro problems call mostly for study of micro situations. The contexts are different, the action is different, the understandings are different. The ideas of qualitative inquiry are of value in both.

Most qualitative research focuses on the microsituation, the ordinary dog-bites-man situation, where the carefully collected personal experiences of people and dogs observed take on meaning through past experiences of the people doing the observing.

> The task is not so much to see what no one yet has seen, but to think what no body yet has thought about what everyone sees. (Arthur Schopenhauer, 1818, quoted in Athena McLean and Annette Leibing, 2000, p. 20)

And then writing it up so that readers have something of a vicarious experience. So much more is learned by seeing that experience close up than by finding it in distanced sources.

If you prefer a more disciplined retrospective for this book, you may turn back again to Box 1.2 in the first chapter. But you and I have spent a lot of time together, and I thought we might just sit here and think about this while we still have some time together. So. . . .

Glossary
Meanings for This Book

I have never found a concept that was grasped in a word.
—JACQUES DERRIDA (2005)

action research: a study of one's own practice.

adroitly: cleverly.

advance organizer: orientation of a reader's mind to think certain things.

advocacy: support, a championing of.

aggregative: collected numerically.

amatory: affection stirring.

ameliorate: to make better.

analysis: act of carefully taking apart.

apocryphal: untrue but having moral force.

assertion: something said with force.

attributes: descriptive words, variables.

attribution: a specification of the cause.

bailiwick: a home place.

binocular resolution: depth perception.

box: virtual storage for a topical collection of knowledge.

commonality: something shared together, held in common.

computer-enhanced: assisted by a computer.

concept: a mental interpretation generalized from instances.

constructivist view: belief that reality is more what we presume than what it is.

content: foreground information, substantive knowledge.

context: background information.

convergence: narrowing to the most important things to say.

coordinate: partnered.

correspondence: acting similarly.

counterintuitive: against common sense.

criterial thinking: thinking that reality should be represented by scalar descriptions.

data set: a group of data, perhaps in a tape, a record of observation, a description, a story, all responses to one question, all data under one code, etc.

data source: the place or people from which we get the information.

declarative: stating something as a fact.

deconstruct: to question the values.

decontextualized: removed from its contexts.

dialectic: logical argumentation to resolve two opposing ideas.

didactic: telling it directly.

disaggregation: taking apart.

duality: two-sided, polar opposites.

element: a tiny building block.

elementalistic: high concentration on the parts.

ellipse: an oval.

embedded case: a small case included in the study of a larger case; a minicase.

embraceable: able to get a hold of.

emic issues: contending arguments held among those at the research site.

empathic: feeling connected with other persons distressed or emotionally beset.

empirical: based on sensory experiences.

entrapment: steering the talk into revelations.

enumeration: counting.

epiphany: brilliant insight.

episodic: happenings at certain times.

epistemology: understanding of what knowledge is.

ethnographic: cultural observations.

etic issues: contending arguments realized by the researcher.

evaluand: the thing evaluated.

exhibit question: an interview question including a picture or selection of text about which the question is asked.

experiential knowing: to know something by experiencing it.

experimentalism: belief in learning by conducting experiments.

explication: something stated carefully and with precision.

field (as in fieldwork): going to where the action is.

field (as in field oriented): attention to a research discipline, such as music.

forensics: preparing evidence for formal argument, such as in court.

foreshadowing question: a major concern anticipated.

formulaic: looking like it was done mechanically.

fortuitous: determined by chance.

functional relationship: formal statement of how one thing is determined by others.

generalization: applying a statement to many or all cases.

habituation: custom or habit.

haptic: bodily sensation.

Hawthorne effect: effect on outcomes from being given increased attention.

hermeneutics: the study of the meanings of human action.

heuristic: a guide to thinking.

histrionic: theatrical.

holistic: giving attention to the whole more than to one or more parts.

icon: a highly meaningful image.

incrementally: small steps one at a time.

informant: someone on the inside willing to tell you about something.

information domains: topics, content categories.

information set: cluster of data from a method or about a topic.

intellectual structure: any patterning of one's thinking.

interpretive: relies on human reasoning and judgment.

interrogatory: questioning.

interview records: data obtained by questioning, usually face-to-face.

issue: a problematic theme having tension and advocacy.

iterative: deliberately repetitive.

level of confidence: a degree of assurance, sometimes statistically indicated.

logic modeling: the steps of a pattern of correlations.

lore: knowledge from experience.

macroanalysis: the analysis of very large collectivities.

macrocosm: a very big system.

member checking: asking a data source to confirm your reporting.

microanalysis: the close study of small details.

microcosm: a smaller system, sometimes mirroring a larger one.

microethnography: elaborate inquiry into a small group or activity.

minicase: a smaller case within the study of a larger one; an embedded case.

mixed methods: using more than one technique to study one thing.

multiple realities: alternative perspectives.

naturalistic generalization: knowledge from direct experience.

naturalistic research: observation of ordinary happenings in their own places.

noninterventionist: avoiding influencing the ongoing activities.

norm-referencing: comparing an individual to a group of individuals.

objective thinking: relying on impersonal measurement.

observations: data collected, especially by watching.

pantheon: a panel of special people.

participant observation: the researcher joins the activity under study to learn more of the experience.

participatory research: when the people studied help to run the research.

particularization: attending to what is important about the cases at hand.

patch: a story, some text, or other item potentially worthy of inclusion in the report.

patronizing: providing service to.

pattern: a repetition of marks or activity seen as a model for identification.

petite generalization: a finding expected to hold under quite similar conditions.

phenomena: similar happenings experienced.

phenomenological: reality known through sensory experience.

phronesis: strategic, grand, explanatory, judicious knowledge.

placebo: a pretend treatment.

plagiarism: falsely using the writing of someone else as your own.

prequestions: preliminary questions.

probative evidence: evidence that proves a point.

progressive focusing: redirecting the study along the way.

protocol: a data-gathering procedure.

qualifying examination: a comprehensive predissertation test.

quintain: a theme or research question running through multiple cases.

reconnoitering: pausing to reconsider the way to go.

redundancy: repetition.

relativistic: deciding on the basis of the immediate circumstances.

research: deliberate study, inquiry, a seeking to know.

research question: statement of the aim of the research.

rival hypothesis: an alternative explanation.

rubric: a rule or checklist for evaluating something.

scalar: using measurements.

semistructured interview: a set of questions, asked the same of all, easily coded.

sequence: a continuous or connected series, one thing after another.

situationality: the idea that meanings are influenced by surrounding contexts.

societal: for the social system as a whole.

stakeholder: someone who stands to lose if the thing doesn't work.

stricture: limit, constraint, prohibition.

structural thinking: formalistic thinking, as with order, lists, categories.

subjective thinking: thinking based on one's own values.

substantive: pertaining to the subject matter content or knowledge.

survey information: data obtained by asking a standardized set of questions.

synthesis: putting the parts together to make a whole.

techne: technical knowledge, knowing how to do it.

tendrils: stems.

theme: a topic or focus of interest within the research.

thick description: theory-based description emphasizing the experience of those studied.

topic: subject matter or a focus of interest within the research.

transformative: life changing.

traumatic: hurtful.

trepidation: fear.

triangulation: using additional data to check or expand one's interpretations.

ubiquitous: happening everywhere.

vicarious experience: experiencing through someone else's direct experience.

visceral: instinctual rather than intellectual awareness.

workable: a detailed story of human activity useful for refining a concept.

Bibliography

Nicholas Abercrombie, Stephen Hill, and Bryan Turner, 1984. *Dictionary of sociology.* London: Penguin Books.

Patricia Adler and Peter Adler, 1994. Observation techniques. In Norman Denzin and Yvonna Lincoln, editors, *Handbook of qualitative research.* Thousand Oaks, CA: Sage.

Michael Agar, 1980. *The professional stranger.* New York: Academic Press.

Reginald Arkell, 1916. *All the rumours.* London: Duckworth & Co.

David Ausubel, 1963. *The psychology of meaningful verbal learning.* New York: Grune & Stratton.

Stephen Baker, 2008. *The numerati.* New York: Houghton-Mifflin.

John Bartlett, 1968. *Bartlett's familiar quotations.* 14th edition. Boston: Little, Brown.

Howard Becker, 1998. *Tricks of the trade.* Chicago: University of Chicago Press.

Howard Becker, Blanche Geer, Everett Hughes, and Anselm Strauss, 1961. *Boys in white: Student culture in medical school.* Chicago: University of Chicago Press.

Leonard Bickman and Debra Rog, editors, 1998. *Handbook of applied social research methods.* Thousand Oaks, CA: Sage.

Henry Black, Joseph Nolan, and Jacqueline Nolan-Haley, editors, 1990. *Black's law dictionary*, sixth edition. St. Paul, MN: West.

William Blake, 1982a. Annotations to Sir Joshua Reynolds's "Disclosures." In David Erdman, editor, *The complete poetry and prose of William Blake.* Los Angeles and Berkeley: University of California Press. (Original work published 1808)

William Blake, 1982b. The everlasting Gospel. In David Erdman, editor, *The complete poetry and prose of William Blake*. Los Angeles and Berkeley: University of California Press.

William Blake, 1997. In Walter Feldman, editor, *Auguries of innocence*. Ziggurat Press (Library of Congress).

Ingwer Borg and Patrick Groenen, 2005. *Modern multidimensional scaling: Theory and applications*. New York: Springer.

Kathryn Borman, 1984. *Fitting into a job*. Columbus: Ohio State University.

Paul Bourdieu, 1992. The practice of reflective sociology (the Paris Workshop). In Paul Bourdieu and L. J. D. Wacquant, editors, *An invitation to reflexive sociology*. Chicago: University of Chicago Press.

Ivan Brady, 2006. Poetics for a planet. In Norman Denzin and Yvonna Lincoln, editors, *Handbook of qualitative research*, third edition. Thousand Oaks, CA: Sage.

Ian Brown, 2006. Nurses' attitudes towards adult patients who are obese: Literature review. *Journal of Advanced Nursing*, 53(2), 221–232.

Ian Brown and Aitkaterini Psarou, 2007. Literature review of nursing practice in managing obesity in primary care: Developments in the UK. *Journal of Clinical Nursing*, 17(1), 17–28.

Lucy Candib, 1995. *Medicine and the family: A feminist perspective*. New York: Basic Books.

Bruce Chatwin, 1987. *The songlines*. New York: Elizabeth Sifton Books.

Eleanor Chelimsky, 2007. Factors influencing the choice of methods in federal evaluation practice. In George Julnes and Debra Rog, editors, *Informing federal policies on evaluation methodology: Building the evidence base for method choice in government-sponsored evaluation*. San Francisco: Jossey-Bass.

Robert Coles, 1967. *Children of crisis*. Boston: Little, Brown.

Robert Coles, 1989. *The call of stories: Teaching and the moral imagination*. New York: Houghton Mifflin.

Thomas Cook, 2006. *Using experiments as a causal gold standard to demonstrate that they are not unique as a causal gold standard*. Keynote address presented at the meeting of the Eastern Evaluation Research Society, Abescon, NJ, April.

John Craig, 1993. *The nature of co-operation*. Cheektowaga, NY: Black Rose Books.

John Creswell and Vicki Plano Clark, 2006. *Designing and conducting mixed methods research*. Thousand Oaks, CA: Sage.

Lee Cronbach, 1974. *Beyond the two disciplines of scientific psychology*. Address presented at the annual meeting of the American Psychological Association, September 2, New Orleans, LA.

Sara Delamont, 1992. *Fieldwork in educational settings*. London: Academic Press.

Terry Denny, 1978. *In defense of story telling as a first step in educational research*. Paper presented at the annual meeting of the International Reading Association, Houston, TX, May.

Norman Denzin, 1989. *The research act*, third edition. Upper Saddle River, NJ: Prentice Hall.

Norman Denzin, 2001. *Interpretive interactionism.* Thousand Oaks, CA: Sage.

Norman Denzin, 2002. *Pedagogy, politics, and ethics.* Thousand Oaks, CA: Sage.

Norman Denzin and Michael Giardina, 2008. *Qualitative inquiry and the politics of evidence.* Walnut Creek, CA: Left Coast Press.

Norman Denzin and Yvonna Lincoln, editors, 1994. *Handbook of qualitative research.* Thousand Oaks, CA: Sage

Norman Denzin and Yvonna Lincoln, editors, 2000. *Handbook of qualitative research*, second edition. Thousand Oaks, CA: Sage

Norman Denzin and Yvonna Lincoln, editors, 2006. *Handbook of qualitative research*, third edition. Thousand Oaks, CA: Sage

Jacques Derrida, 2005. *Paper machine.* Palo Alto, CA: Stanford University Press.

William Dilthey, 1910. *The construction of the historical world of the human studies (Der Aufbauder Welt in den Geisteswissenshchaften). Gesammelte Schriften I–VII.* Leipzig, Germany: Teubner.

Ivan Doig, 1980. *Winter brothers: A season at the edge of America.* New York: Harcourt Brace.

Michael Duneier, 1992. *Slim's table.* Chicago: University of Chicago Press.

Svitlana Efimova and Natalia Sofiy, 2004. *Inclusive education: The Step by Step Program influencing children, teachers, parents and state policies in Ukraine.* Noncirculated document. Budapest: Open Society Institute. Reprinted in Robert Stake, 2006, *Multiple case study analysis.* New York: Guilford Press.

Elliot Eisner, 1991. *The enlightened eye.* New York: Macmillan.

Ralph Waldo Emerson, 1850. *Representative men.* Oxford, UK: Smith, Elder.

Ralph Waldo Emerson, 1860. Worship. In *The conduct of life.* Oxford, UK: Smith, Elder.

Robert Emerson, 2004. Working with "key incidents." In Clive Seale, Giampietro Gobo, Jaber Gubrium, and David Silverman, editors, *Qualitative research practice.* Thousand Oaks, CA: Sage.

Kadriye Ercikan, 2008. Limitations in sample-to-population generalizing. In Kadriye Ercikan and Wolff-Michael Roth, editors, *Generalizing from educational research: Beyond qualitative and quantitative polarization.* London: Taylor & Francis.

Kadriye Ercikan and Wolff-Michael Roth, editors, 2008. *Generalizing from educational research: Beyond qualitative and quantitative polarization.* London: Taylor & Francis.

Frederick Erickson, 1986. Qualitative methods in research on teaching. In Merlin Wittrock, editor, *Handbook of research on teaching*, third edition. New York: Macmillan.

Frederick Erickson, 2008. Four points concerning policy-oriented qualitative research. In Norman Denzin and Michael Giardina, editors, *Qualita-*

tive inquiry and the politics of evidence. Walnut Creek, CA: Left Coast Press.

Ned Flanders, 1970. *Analyzing teaching behavior.* New York: Addison-Wesley.

Uwe Flick, 2002. *An introduction to qualitative research.* London: Sage.

Bent Flyvbjerg, 2001. *Making social science matter* (translated by S. Sampson). Cambridge, UK: Cambridge University Press.

Bent Flyvbjerg, 2004. Five misunderstandings about case-study research. In Clive Seale, Giampietro Gobo, Jaber Gubrium, and David Silverman, editors, *Qualitative research practice.* London: Sage.

Arthur Foshay, 1993. *Action research: An early history in the United States.* Paper presented at the annual meeting of the American Educational Research Association, April.

R. H. Franke and J. D. Kaul, 1978. The Hawthorne experiments: First statistical interpretation. *American Sociological Review, 43,* 623–643.

Rita Frerichs, 2002. *The producer guild.* Urbana: Center for Instructional Research and Curriculum Evaluation, University of Illinois.

Gabriel García Márquez, 1970. *One hundred years of solitude.* New York: Harper & Row.

Clifford Geertz, 1983. *Local knowledge: Further essays in interpretive anthropology.* New York: Basic Books.

Clifford Geertz, 1988. *Works and lives: The anthropologist as author.* Palo Alto: Stanford University Press.

Clifford Geertz, 1993. *Thick description: Toward an interpretive theory of culture.* New York: Fontana.

Barney Glaser and Anselm Strauss, 1967. *The discovery of grounded theory: Strategies for qualitative research.* Chicago: Aldine.

Jennifer Greene, 1996. Qualitative evaluation and scientific citizenship: Reflections and refractions. *Evaluation, 2,* 277–289.

Jennifer Greene, 1997. Participatory evaluation. *Advances in Program Evaluation, 3,* 171–189.

Jennifer Greene, 2007. *Mixed methods in social inquiry.* San Francisco: Jossey-Bass.

Markus Grutsch, 2001. *From responsive to collaborative evaluation.* Unpublished doctoral dissertation, University of Innsbruck, Austria.

Amy Gutman, 1999. *Democratic education.* Princeton, NJ: Princeton University Press.

David Halberstam, 2007. *The coldest winter.* New York: Hall.

Bent Hamer, writer/director, and Jörgen Bergmark, writer, 2003. *Kitchen stories* [Motion picture]. Sweden: ICA Projects.

David Hamilton, no date. *In search of structure: Essays from an open plan school* [Mimeograph]. Edinburgh, UK: Scottish Council for Research in Education.

Ian Hodder, 1994. The interpretation of documents and material culture. In Norman Denzin and Yvonna Lincoln, editors, *Handbook of qualitative research.* Thousand Oaks, CA: Sage.

Ernest House, 1980. *Evaluating with validity.* Thousand Oaks, CA: Sage.

Ernest House, 2006. *Democracy and evaluation.* Keynote address presented at the biannual meeting of the European Evaluation Society, Berlin, Germany, October.

Ernest House and Kenneth Howe, 1999. *Values in evaluation and social research.* Thousand Oaks, CA: Sage.

Burke Johnson and Larry Christensen, 2008. *Educational research: Quantitative, qualitative, and mixed approaches,* third edition. Thousand Oaks, CA: Sage.

Iván Jorrín-Abellán, 2006. *Formative portrayals emerged from a Computer Supported Collaborative Learning environment: A case study.* Unpublished doctoral dissertation [in Spanish], College of Education and Social Work, Department of Pedagogy, University of Valladolid, Spain.

Iván Jorrín-Abellán. 2008. Personal communication.

Anthony Kelly and Robert Yin, 2007. Strengthening structured abstracts for education research: The need for claim-based structured abstracts. *Educational Researcher, 36*(3), 133–138.

Diana Kelly-Byrne, 1989. *A child's play life: An ethnographic study.* New York: Teachers College Press.

Stephen Kemmis, 2007. "Here." Personal communication.

Stephen Kemmis and Matts Mattsson, 2007. Praxis-related research: Serving two masters? *Pedagogy, Culture, and Society, 15*(2), 185–214.

Stephen Kemmis and Robin McTaggart, 2006. Participative action research. In Norman Denzin and Yvonna Lincoln, editors, *Handbook of qualitative research,* third edition. Thousand Oaks, CA: Sage.

A. L. Kennedy, 1999. *On bullfighting.* New York: Random House.

Mary Kennedy, 2007. Defining a literature. *Educational Researcher, 36*(3), 139–147.

Eva Koncoková and Jana Handzelová, 2004. *Impact of Step by Step at the Roma settlement Jarovnice-Karice: Slovakia community resource mobilization.* Budapest: Open Society Institute.

Jonathan Kozol, 1992. *Savage inequities.* New York: Harper Perennial.

Antjie Krog, 2009. " . . . *if it means he gets his humanity back . . .* ": *The worldview underpinning the South African Truth and Reconciliation Commission.* Keynote address presented at the Fifth International Congress of Qualitative Inquiry, University of Illinois at Urbana-Champaign, May 20.

Milan Kundera, 1984. *The unbearable lightness of being.* New York: Harper & Row.

Akira Kurosawa, director, 1951. *Rashomon* [Motion picture]. Japan: Daiei Motion Picture Company.

Saville Kushner, 1992. *A musical education: Innovation in the conservatoire.* East Geelong, Australia: Deakin University Press.

Saville Kushner, 2008. *Chair's introduction.* Paper presented at the United Kingdom Evaluation Society Annual Conference, Bristol, October.

Ellen Condliffe Lagemann, 2002. *An elusive science: The troubling history of educational research.* Chicago: University of Chicago Press.

Haldor Laxness, 1968. *Under the glacier*. Reykjavik, Iceland: Vaka-Helgafell.

Raymond Lee, 2000. *Unobtrusive methods in social research*. Milton Keynes, UK: Open University Press.

You-Jin Lee, 2008. Personal communication.

Annette Leibing and Athena McLean, 2000. "Learn to value your shadow!" An introduction to the margins of fieldwork. In Athena McLean and Annette Leibing, editors, *The shadow side of fieldwork: Exploring the blurred borders between ethnography and life*. Chichester, UK: Blackwell.

Elliot Leibow, 1967. *Talley's corner*. Boston: Little, Brown.

Kurt Lewin, Ronald Lippitt, and Ralph White, 1939. Patterns of aggressive behavior in an experimentally created social climate. *Journal of Social Psychology*, 10, 271–301.

Oscar Lewis, 1966. *La vida*. New York: Random House.

Sarah Lightfoot, 1983. *The good high school*. New York: Basic Books.

Mark Lipsey and David Cordray, 2000. Evaluation methods for social intervention. *Annual Review of Psychology*, 51, 345–375.

Donileen Loseke and Spencer Cahill, 2004. Publishing qualitative manuscripts: Lessons learned. In Clive Seale, Giampietro Gobo, Jaber Gubrium, and David Silverman, editors, *Qualitative research practice*. London: Sage.

Linda Mabry, 1991. Nicole, seeking attention. In *Students who fail*. Bloomington, IN: Phi Delta Kappa.

Barry MacDonald and Rob Walker, 1977. Case study and the social philosophy of educational research. In David Hamilton, David Jenkins, Christina King, Barry MacDonald, and Malcolm Parlett, editors, *Beyond the numbers game*. London: Macmillan.

John Mackie, 1974. *The cement of the universe: A study of causation*. Oxford, UK: Clarendon Press.

Bronislaw Malinowski, 1984. *Argonauts of the Western Pacific*. Prospect Heights, IL: Waveland Press. (Original work published 1922)

George Marcus, 2003. On the unbearable slowness of being an anthropologist now. *Cross-Cultural Poetics*, 12, 7.

Annette Markham, 2004. The Internet as research context. In Clive Seale, Giampietro Gobo, Jaber Gubrium, and David Silverman, editors, *Qualitative research practice*. London: Sage.

Barry McGaw, 2007. *International comparisons of quality*. Paper presented at the annual meeting of the American Educational Research Association, Chicago, April.

Michele McIntosh and Janice Morse, 2008. Institutional review boards and the ethics of emotion. In Norman Denzin and Michael Giardina, editors, *Qualitative inquiry and the politics of evidence*. Walnut Creek, CA: Left Coast Press.

John McPhee, 1966. *The headmaster*. New York: Farrar, Strauss, & Giroux.

Sharon Merriam, 2009. *Qualitative research*. San Francisco: Jossey-Bass.

Donna Mertens and Pauline Ginsberg, 2008. *The handbook of social research ethics*. Thousand Oaks, CA: Sage.

Matthew Miles and Michael Huberman, 1984. *Qualitative data analysis: A sourcebook of new methods.* Thousand Oaks, CA: Sage.

John Stuart Mill, 1984. A system of logic: Ratiocinative and inductive. New York: Longmans, Green. (Original work published 1843)

Robert Mislevy, Pamela Moss, and James Gee, 2008. On qualitative and quantitative reasoning in validity. In Kadriye Ercikan and Wolff-Michael Roth, editors, *Generalizing from educational research: Beyond qualitative and quantitative polarization.* London: Taylor & Francis.

John Moffitt, 1961. To look at any thing. In *The Living Seed.* Orlando, FL: Houghton Mifflin Harcourt.

Juny Montoya, 2004. Responsive and democratic evaluation of a law school curriculum: A case study. Doctoral dissertation (Urbana, IL: University of Illinois).

Juny Montoya Vargas, 2008. *The case for active learning in legal education: An evaluative case study of the curriculum reform at Los Andes University.* Saarbrücken, Germany: VDM Verlag Dr. Müller Aktiengesellschaft & Co. KG.

April Munson, 2009. Personal communication.

Joseph Novak, Retrieved September 1, 2008. *Concept maps: What the heck is this?* [Excerpted, rearranged, and annotated from an online manuscript.] www.msu.edu/~luckie/ctools/.

Joseph Novak and Bob Gowin, 1984. *Learning how to learn.* Cambridge, UK: Cambridge University Press.

Malcolm Parlett and David Hamilton, 1977. Evaluation as illumination: A new approach to the study of innovatory programmes. In David Hamilton, David Jenkins, Christina King, Barry MacDonald, and Malcolm Parlett, editors, *Beyond the numbers game.* London: Macmillan.

Michael Patton, 1997. *Utilization-focused evaluation.* Thousand Oaks, CA: Sage.

Ivan Pavlov, 1936. *Bequest to the academic youth of Soviet Russia.* Quoted in John Bartlett, *Bartlett's familiar quotations,* 14th edition (p. 818). Boston: Little, Brown.

Alan Peshkin, 1986. *God's choice.* Chicago: University of Chicago Press.

Michael Polanyi, 1958. *Personal knowledge.* New York: Harper & Row.

Michael Polanyi, 1966. *The tacit dimension.* New York: Doubleday.

Pierre Poreieu, 1990. The scholastic point of view. *Cultural Anthropology, 5,* 380–391.

Lindsay Prior, 2004. Documents. In Clive Seale, Giampietro Gobo, Jaber Gubrium, and David Silverman, editors, *Qualitative research practice.* London: Sage.

Paul Rabinow, 2008. *Marking time.* Princeton, NJ: Princeton University Press.

Luisa Rosu, 2009. Thinking and creativity in learning mathematics teaching. Doctoral dissertation. Urbana, IL: University of Illinois.

Wolff-Michael Roth, 2008. Phenomenological and dialectical perspectives on the relation between the general and the particular. In Kadriye Ercikan and Wolff-Michael Roth, editors, *Generalizing from educational research: Beyond qualitative and quantitative polarization.* London: Taylor & Francis.

Anne Ryen, 2004. Ethical issues. In Clive Seale, Giampietro Gobo, Jaber Gubrium, and David Silverman, editors, *Qualitative research practice.* London: Sage.

Harvey Sacks, 1984. On doing "being ordinary." In J. M. Atkinson and J. Heritage, editors, *Structures of social action: Studies in conversational analysis.* Cambridge, UK: Cambridge University Press.

William Saroyan, 1972. *Places where I've done time.* New York: Praeger.

Donald Schön, 1983. *The reflective practitioner: How professionals think in action.* New York: Basic Books.

Arthur Schopenhauer, 1818. The world as will and representation. Quoted in "Learn to love your shadow!" In Athena McLean and Annette Leibing, editors, An introduction to the margins of fieldwork, 2000, *The shadow side of fieldwork: Exploring the blurred areas between ethnography and life* (p. 20). Chichester, UK: Blackwell.

Thomas Schwandt, 1997. *Qualitative inquiry: A dictionary of terms.* Thousand Oaks, CA: Sage.

Michael Scriven, 1976. Maximizing the power of causal investigation. The *modus operandi* method. In Gene Glass, editor, *Evaluation Studies Review Annual,* Volume 1. Thousand Oaks, CA: Sage.

Michael Scriven, 1994. The final synthesis. *Evaluation Practice,* 15(3), 367–382.

Michael Scriven, 1998. Bias. In Rita Davis, editor, *Proceedings of the Stake Symposium on Educational Evaluation* (Champaign, Illinois, May 8–9, 1998.) Urbana, IL: Center for Instructional Research and Curriculum Evaluation, College of Education, University of Illinois.

Clive Seale, Giampietro Gobo, Jaber Gubrium, and David Silverman, editors, 2004. *Qualitative research practice.* London: Sage.

Thomas Seals, 1985. *A theoretical construction of gender issues in marital therapy.* Unpublished doctoral dissertation, University of Illinois.

Walênia Silva, 2007. *Urban music: A case study of communities of learning in a music school.* Unpublished doctoral dissertation, University of Illinois.

David Silverman, 2000. *Doing qualitative research.* London: Sage.

David Silverman, 2007. *A very short, fairly interesting and reasonably cheap book about qualitative research.* London: Sage.

Finbarr Sloane, 2008. Comments on Slavin: Through the looking glass: Experiments, quasi-experiments, and the medical model. *Educational Researcher,* 37(1), 41–46.

Linda Tuhiwai Smith, 2005. *On tricky ground: Researching the native in the Age of Uncertainty.* Keynote address presented at the Congress of Qualitative Inquiry, Urbana, IL, May 5.

Louis Smith, 2008. The culture of Cambridge: Found and constructed. *Perspectives in Education,* 24(4), 197–220.

Louis Smith and William Geoffrey, 1968. *The complexities of an urban classroom: An analysis toward a general theory of teaching.* New York: Holt, Rinehart, & Winston.

Terry Solomonson, 2005. Corps values: A case study. Urbana, IL: Center for Instructional Research and Curriculum Evaluation, College of Education, University of Illinois.

Robert Stake, 1961. Learning parameters, aptitudes, and achievements. *Psychometric Monographs*, no. 9. Richmond, VA: Psychometric Society.

Robert Stake, 1986. *Quieting reform: Social science and social action in an urban youth program.* Urbana, IL: University of Illinois Press.

Robert Stake, 1995. *The art of case study research.* Thousand Oaks, CA: Sage.

Robert Stake, 2000. Kimberly Grogan, a newly affiliated teacher. In Robert Stake and Marya Burke, 2000. Evaluating teaching. (An evaluation report) Urbana, IL: Center for Instructional Research and Curriculum Evaluation, College of Education, University of Illinois.

Robert Stake, 2006. *Multiple case study analysis.* New York: Guilford Press.

Robert Stake, Lizanne DeStefano, Delwyn Harnisch, Kathryn Sloane, and Rita Davis, 1997. *Evaluation of the National Youth Sports Program.* Urbana, IL: Center for Instructional Research and Curriculum Evaluation, College of Education, University of Illinois.

Robert Stake and Jack Easley, 1978. *Case studies in science education.* Urbana, IL: Center for Instructional Research and Curriculum Evaluation, College of Education, University of Illinois.

Robert Stake, William Platt, Rita Davis, Neil Vanderveen, and Khalil Dirani, 2003. *Integrating Veterans Benefits Association training and evaluation.* Urbana, IL: Center for Instructional Research and Curriculum Evaluation, College of Education, University of Illinois.

Robert Stake and Deborah Trumbull, 1982. Naturalistic generalizations. *Review Journal of Philosophy and Social Science*, 7, 1–12.

Anselm Strauss and Juliet Corbin, 1990. *Basics of qualitative research: Grounded theory procedures and techniques.* Thousand Oaks, CA: Sage.

Daniel Stufflebeam, 1968. *Evaluation as enlightenment for decision making.* Columbus, OH: Evaluation Center, Ohio State University.

Daniel Stufflebeam, 1971. The relevance of the CIPP evaluation model for educational accountability. *Journal of Research and Development in Education, 1*, 19–25.

Daniel Stufflebeam and Anthony Shinkfield, 2007. *Theories, approaches, and practices of evaluation.* Thousand Oaks, CA: Sage.

Sun Yat-Sen, 1986. *Chung-shan Ch'uan-shu* [*The complete works of Sun Yat-Sen*, Volume II]. Beijing: Chung Hwa.

Louis (Studs) Terkel, 1975. *Working: People talk about what they do all day and how they feel about what they do.* New York: Avon.

Joseph Tobin, David Wu, and Dana Davidson, 1991. *Preschool in three cultures: Japan, China, and the United States.* New Haven, CT: Yale University Press.

Leo Tolstoy, 1978. *War and peace* (translated by Rosemary Edmonds). London: Penguin. (Original work published 1869)

William Trochim, 1989. Concept mapping: Soft science or hard art? *Evaluation and Program Planning, 12*, 87–110.

Megan Tschannen-Moran and Wayne Hoy, 2000. A multidisciplinary analysis of the nature, meaning, and measurement of trust. *Review of Educational Research, 70*(4), 547–593.

Ralph Turner and Lewis Killian, 1987. *Collective behavior.* Englewood Cliffs, NJ: Prentice Hall.

John van Maanen, 1988. *Tales of the field: On writing ethnography.* Chicago: University of Chicago Press.

Georg Hendrik von Wright, 1971. *Explanation and understanding.* Ithaca, NY: Cornell University Press.

Rob Walker, 1978. Case studies in science education: Boston. In Robert Stake and John Easley, editors, *Case Studies in Science Education.* Urbana, IL: Center for Instructional Research and Curriculum Evaluation, University of Illinois.

Robert Walker, Lesley Hoggart, and Gayle Hamilton, 2008. Random assignment and informed consent: A case study of multiple perspectives. *American Journal of Evaluation, 29*, 156–174.

James Watson, 1969. *The double helix.* London: Signet Books.

Eugene Webb, Donald Campbell, R. D. Schwartz, and Lee Sechrest, 1966. *Unobtrusive methods: Nonreactive research in the social sciences.* Chicago: Rand McNally.

Aaron Wildavsky, 1995. *But is it true?* Cambridge, MA: Harvard University Press.

Jerry Willis, 2009. *Qualitative research methods in education and educational technology.* New York: Information Age.

Harry Wolcott, 1973. *The man in the principal's office: An ethnography.* New York: Holt, Rinehart, & Winston.

Robert K. Yin, 1981. The case study as a serious research strategy. *Knowledge: Creation, Diffusion, Utilization, 3*, 97–114.

Mandawuy (formerly Bakamana) Yunupingu, 1991. A plan for Ganma research. In Rhonda Bunbury, Warren Hastings, John Henry, and Robin McTaggart, editors, *Aboriginal pedagogy: Aboriginal teachers speak out* (pp. 98–106). East Geelong, Australia: Deakin University Press.

Author Index

Subject Index

Page numbers followed by an *f* or a *t* indicate figures or tables.

About the Author

Robert E. Stake, PhD, is director of the Center for Instructional Research and Curriculum Evaluation at the University of Illinois at Urbana-Champaign. He is one of several educational researchers who created theory and practice for educational program evaluation in the 1960s. His responsive evaluation approach emphasizes the study of classroom experience, personal interaction, and institutional processes and contexts, often in the form of case studies. Among the evaluative studies he has directed are studies in science and arts education; model programs; and conventional teaching, including higher education, special education and, with Bernadine Evans Stake, gender equity. He is the author of *Quieting Reform: Social Science and Social Action in an Urban Youth Program* (1986) about Charles Murray's evaluation of Cities-in-Schools and four other books on research methodology: *Multiple Case Study Analysis* (2006); *Standards-Based and Responsive Evaluation* (2003); *the Art of Case Study Research* (1995); and *Evaluating the Arts in Education: A Responsive Approach* (1975). In 1988, he received the Lazarsfeld Award from the American Evaluation Association for his evaluation work, and the Presidential Citation from the American Educational Research Association in 2007. He holds honorary doctorates from the University of Uppsala, Sweden, and the University of Valladolid, Spain. For many years, he has been a prominent voice in a transatlantic "invisible college" of like-minded evaluators questioning contexts and conventions for educational evaluation and infusing evaluation with fairness and a valuing of experience.